Clinical Embryology

MONOGRAPHS FOR STUDENTS OF MEDICINE

SERIES EDITORS

Professor R. J. Harrison, F.R.S., M.D., D.Sc.,
School of Anatomy, University of Cambridge, Cambridge

Dr. A. W. Asscher, M.D., F.R.C.P.
K.R.U.F. Institute of Renal Disease, Welsh National School of Medicine, Cardiff

AN OUTLINE OF GERIATRICS by Dr. M. Hodkinson
THE HUMAN HEART AND CIRCULATION by Dr. V. Navaratnam
GENERAL PRACTICE FOR STUDENTS OF MEDICINE by Dr. R. Harvard Davis
COMPARATIVE PLACENTATION: Essays in Structure and Function by Dr. D. Steven
SEX AND INFERTILITY by Professor R. G. Harrison and Mr. C. de Boer
THE PATHOGENESIS OF INFECTIOUS DISEASE by Professor C. A. Mims
CLINICAL EMBRYOLOGY by Professor R. G. Harrison

MONOGRAPHS FOR STUDENTS OF MEDICINE

CLINICAL EMBRYOLOGY

R. G. HARRISON, M.A., D.M.

Derby Professor of Anatomy, University of Liverpool

1978

ACADEMIC PRESS

London   New York   San Francisco

A Subsidiary of Harcourt Brace Jovanovich, Publishers

ACADEMIC PRESS (LONDON) LTD.
24-28 Oval Road,
London, NW1

United States Edition published by
ACADEMIC PRESS INC.
111 Fifth Avenue
New York, New York 10003

Library of Congress Catalog Card Number: 77-92822
ISBN: 0-12-327840-6

PRINTED IN GREAT BRITAIN BY THE LAVENHAM PRESS LIMITED
LAVENHAM SUFFOLK

Preface

This book is a logical extension of my original Textbook of Human Embryology, now out of print. Any acknowledgments for assistance and the use of illustrations in that book therefore apply equally to this. Since a knowledge of development is becoming increasingly important in the comprehension of anomalies and the surgery of congenital deformities, I have been urged by students to write a completely new book to assist both undergraduates and postgraduates. It is hoped that the undergraduate will find it useful as an adjunct to his clinical studies, just as much as a primer of human development during his preclinical studies of anatomy.

The main aim of this book is to facilitate comprehension of human development as a science which can, in its turn, assist understanding of adult human anatomy, and is therefore designed for the medical student. In addition, the aetiology of developmental defects and the role of embryology in disease is also discussed in each chapter in a section on Clinical Relationships. In this way, therefore, the text will be found useful by clinical students and postgraduates. The postgraduate revising anatomy for certain examinations, such as the primary F.R.C.S., will also find it necessary to understand the developmental features of each region.

Much morphological embryological detail has been omitted and accent placed rather on function. In addition, it has been considered more important to comprehend the nature and features of developmental processes rather than to detail when they occur. The times of developmental events have largely been omitted, since they mostly occur in the first eight weeks anyway, and to be able to recite a long list of dates within that period serves no useful purpose.

There is some diversity of opinion as to what features of embryology should be taught, and to what extent. It is hoped, however, that detail has not been neglected too much for the majority of medical schools and that the text is sufficiently readable although concise.

Liverpool,   R. G. HARRISON
January 1978

Contents

1

Introduction

Apart from its value as an academic discipline, the study of human embryology is of great practical importance, since without a thorough knowledge of it a proper comprehension of adult human anatomy and of many aspects of the clinical sciences of obstetrics and gynaecology is impossible.

Human embryology is concerned with the development of the human being, the term "development" being defined as the continuous modification of an individual's total life processes which transpire between the egg stage and the adult form. This progressive process is to be distinguished from physiological activities in that it mainly produces a slow change in form, whereas in the usually rapid physiological activities the basic form remains unaltered and stable. Embryological events prevail in the prenatal period; therefore they have been considered "preparatory" in nature and purpose has even been imputed. Such *teleological* explanations are seldom warranted, since it is often impossible to know the outcome of certain embryological processes, and purpose cannot be ascribed to a process whose outcome is unknown.

The term *ontogeny* is used to describe the series of successive stages during the development of an individual. Because of its resemblance to *phylogeny,* the series of stages of modification in shape of *adult* animals in successive generations during evolution, attempts were made in the nineteenth century to correlate the two. In 1828 von Baer proposed very important laws relating phylogeny to ontogeny (see de Beer, 1958), the most important of which proclaimed that man during his development resembles the *embryos* of more lowly vertebrates.

The morphological characteristics of man are produced during development by interaction between internal (genetic) factors and external (environmental) ones. Such normal interaction results in a phenotype. The genotype of an individual is the sum total of its genetic constitution. Since there are so many environmental factors essential for the normal development of man it is clear that the genotype cannot determine his phenotype entirely.

Development and differentiation

The process of development involves in itself other independent processes, namely cell division or mitosis, cell migration, growth (that is, augmentation of size) and *differentiation* (see Weiss, 1939, 1953). Development as it affects individual cells implies the production of new characters which make the cell

1

become different first from its own former self, which is the process of growth, and secondly from other cells to which it originally bore resemblance, and this latter process is termed differentiation: in other words, progressive diversification. A fundamental feature of differentiation is that it is incompatible with mitosis, since differentiating tissue shows a decline of relative growth rate. Growth is one of the most fundamental characteristics of development and, of course, it continues in postnatal life as well as occurring prenatally. Figure 1, from the data of His and Russow (see

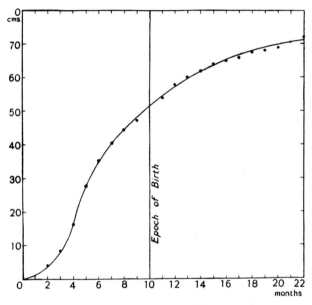

Fig. 1. The curve of human growth (in length or stature) in prenatal and early postnatal life. Composed by Thompson, 1948, from His and Russow's data.

Thompson, 1948), demonstrates that the process of growth of a fetus continues into that of the newborn child. Birth does not, in fact, in itself, produce any marked alteration in this growth, apart from a temporary loss in weight in the immediate postnatal period, which is a well-recognized phenomenon. Figure 2 shows that the velocity of growth of a fetus changes throughout the prenatal period, increasing to a maximum at the fifth month and then gradually decreasing but again merging insensibly at the time of birth into a declining growth rate in the postnatal period up to a certain time (Rao, 1958). In other words, the process of birth itself is merely an incident in the development of a human being, with development, and all that it implies, continuing in the postnatal period.

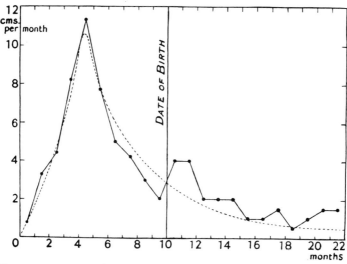

Fig. 2. The mean monthly increments of length or stature in man during prenatal and early postnatal life. Composed by Thompson, 1948, from His and Russow's data.

Organizers

During development individual cells owe their fate to the forces and conditions to which they become subject during the course of this process. One of the most important of such factors is the *organizers*. These were first discovered in the dorsal lip of the amphibian blastopore and it was shown by many experiments that this particular region of the developing amphibian can *induce* neighbouring tissues and so give rise eventually to all essential structures of the embryo. Although the organizers are therefore primarily produced from a relatively small area in the developing embryo, they come to reside in many tissues and in later development may be found in areas rather than specific points. For example, at one stage in development, the notochord and the adjoining paraxial mesoderm together produce organizers which induce the overlying ectoderm to differentiate into the neural tube. There are first of all primary organizers and then secondary organizers causing differentiation in adjoining tissues and these in turn produce tertiary organizers. Many synthetic polycyclic hydrocarbons and compounds of a steroid nature are very active in the induction of tissues (see Needham, 1950). Some oestrogenic hormones, or compounds with oestrogenic activity, for example 1:9-dimethylphenanthrene, are capable of acting as organizers. Certain other compounds which are carcinogenic also have organizer activity, for example 1:2:5:6-dibenzanthracene. Such a relationship is of great importance; the fact that some compounds may effect marked alterations in bodily function and economy or produce neoplasia on the one hand and are also capable of evoking differentiation in the embryo on the other, suggests that certain substances of similar chemical structure are able to exert profound and superficially dissimilar effects on the fate of cells in an organism. The whole process of growth and differentiation of tissues, both normal and abnormal, embryonic and adult, is, therefore, brought into focus and their relationships can be studied at submicroscopic level.

With the more recent discovery of carcinogens which are not hydrocarbons or do not possess a chemical structure of fused ring steroid type, the idea of carcinogenesis resulting from faulty metabolism lost favour in some quarters (see Hieger and Pullinger, 1953). Nevertheless, the fact that such compounds as nitrogen mustard or urethane are able to act as carcinogens does not exclude ultimate carcinogenesis by other substances, since both nitrogen mustard and urethane produce alterations in cell chemistry (see Jacobson, 1958); it is not necessary to hypothesize that compounds become reorganized chemically into a steroid carcinogen, since substances having a carcinogenic action may exert their effect by altering some aspect of cellular activity, such as protein metabolism. Further, tumours and embryos resemble each other in their high aerobic and anaerobic efficiency terms for amino-acid incorporation into their proteins, in contrast to adult mammalian tissue (Quastel and Bickis, 1959). The mechanisms of carcinogenesis have been reviewed by Rous (1959).

Most of the observations on the effects of organizers have been carried out by experimental embryologists who have produced differentiation in host tissues by transplanting grafts from other embryos. By means of such a procedure it is possible to recognize an *evocator*, which is a property of the graft only and initiates histological differentiation, and the *individuator*, which is the property of the graft and the host by means of which the organ tissues are individuated into a system and regional differentiation occurs (Needham, 1950). Inductors which are applied experimentally cause the liberation of evocators from embryonic tissues; several recent experiments point to the protein nature of such evocating substances (see Raven, 1959). When an organizer evokes differentiation, successive processes are involved. For example, in the blastula of an amphibian the cells are plastic and not yet determined. Small pieces of blastula transplanted to other areas of the same blastula or other blastulas produce tissues corresponding to the site into which they are transplanted. During gastrulation, the first manifestation of differentiation is chemo-differentiation, by means of which cells become chemically different from their neighbours. This then advances to a stage of histo-differentiation in which the cells themselves become microscopically different from others; this process is superseded by organogenesis during which the actual organs of the body take shape. At any time during this process, the cells take upon themselves morphological individuality, so that if a piece of gastrula is transplanted into another area of the same gastrula or another gastrula, it will differentiate into what it would have differentiated into anyway before grafting. The existence of organizers has been queried, since it has been claimed that merely pricking certain vertebrate blastulae with a needle initiates "organizer" activity. It may be argued, however, that such mechanical interference would disturb the normal chemical relationships of a cell, so possibly producing evocators from already existing cellular chemical compounds. The development of an organ from a few cells which differentiate in the embryo from a single cell at a particular stage of development is known as "clonal development". For example, a clone of less than ten cells segregates to act as a precursor for the development of the haemopoietic system, the system of the body which forms blood (Wegmann and Gilman, 1970).

There are many relationships of human embryology with other sciences. The fundamental conception of experimental embryology has already been mentioned. The technique of organ or tissue culture using embryonic explants is also utilized for observation of the processes of growth and differentiation of embryonic tissues in isolation. The application of the results of such research to development in the living embryo is very limited, however; the embryonic chick femur in tissue culture reacts very differently from the same bone in the living embryonic chick, since its metabolism is so different. Gaillard (1954), for example, has claimed that it is possible to isolate pieces of human fetal parathyroid in tissue culture and then transplant such pieces of tissue into human beings showing parathyroid insufficiency but not into individuals without such insufficiency. Needham (1931, 1950) and Brachet (1944) have shown that the application of chemistry is essential for the analysis of embryological processes; this is the science of chemical embryology. It should also be remembered that the morphological processes which occur during embryonic life should be considered in relation to their function at any specific time. In other words, embryology should be correlated with physiology at all times and this is the primary aim of functional embryology. The science of histochemistry, by means of which it is possible to observe the chemical characterization of substances in their natural location within cells and tissues (Lison, 1953), has also been utilized to advantage in the study of embryology. For example, Wislocki and Dempsey (1948) have employed histochemical techniques to observe the changes in glycogen, lipoid and other substances in the placenta (see p. 37) during its growth in the human being. Finally, since the developing placenta, to mention only one instance, is capable of producing hormones, embryology is integrally related to endocrinology.

Embryological tissues, like adult tissues, have cells which show pronounced characteristics and it is therefore essential that the student of development should first acquaint himself with the general light and electron microscopic characteristics of the cell (see, for example, Brachet, 1967; Toner and Carr, 1968).

Since development is the basic embryological process, human embryology should not be considered in isolation. Prenatal human development continues into a period of postnatal growth and development, the study of which is yet in its infancy (Tanner, 1962) although occupying more than a quarter of man's lifetime. Ideally, therefore, the study of human embryology should be combined with the study of man himself, anthropology, and must always be correlated with the anatomy of the adult human being.

CLINICAL RELATIONSHIPS

Abnormalities of development produce malformations of adult structure (anomalies) and consequently a sound knowledge of human embryology is essential as a basis for comprehension of human pathology (Willis, 1958). Recently, many observations have been made on the aetiology of anomalies with the knowledge that the administration of certain drugs, for example thalidomide, during pregnancy may result in the production of abnormalities in the offspring. Although some anomalies are genetically determined, it is now realized that certain nutritional deficiencies, hormonal factors, physical and chemical agents and other factors at a given phase of development can produce an anomaly by interfering with the normal embryological process proceeding at that time (see Giroud and Lefebvres, 1957; Kalter and Warkany, 1959; Woollam and Millen, 1960; Woollam, 1967). Certain maternal infections, particularly viruses, such as an attack of rubella (german measles) for example, may have a similar effect. Sever (1967) has claimed that congenital defects occur in the offspring of 20 per cent of the women who have rubella in the first trimester of pregnancy; the risk is greater with infection in the first month. An agent, such as rubella, which produces fetal abnormality, is termed a *teratogen,* and the study of abnormal development and the production of congenital anomalies is known as *teratology.*

Even the subjection of pregnant rats to audio-visual stress (loud noises from bells, buzzers, horns and gongs and flashing lights) is adequate to produce severe developmental anomalies in their offspring (Geber, 1966). Such influences must be exerted in the first three months of pregnancy to have an effect, for it is during this period that differentiation of organs and tissues is proceeding. During the remainder of pregnancy growth of the already established structures is the predominant feature.

It follows, therefore, that teratogenic agents are most likely to exert an effect during the embryonic period of development and it is important to realise that there are many infective, chemical, hormonal, immunological and dietary factors to which the mother may be subjected and which can pass into the circulation of the embryo to affect its development adversely. Maternal age is also a factor; the incidence of anomalies in offspring is much greater in women younger than 17 and older than 35. Thus, the incidence of Down's syndrome (mongolism) is about 25 times greater in a babe born to a woman over 45 years of age. X-rays are also very damaging and for this reason a radiologist may refuse to subject a pregnant woman to therapeutic X-irradiation or take a diagnostic X-ray of her abdomen. It must also be remembered that whilst a deficiency of certain vitamins can be responsible for embryonic anomalies, excessive maternal intake of certain vitamins (e.g. Vitamin A) may have the same effect. There is also considerable evidence that certain anomalies occur particularly in pregnancies which follow a pregnancy ending in a miscarriage or stillbirth.

Such environmental factors are responsible for anomalies of the newborn in about 80% of cases. Only in 20% of birth anomalies can there be recognized a definite genetic basis or chromosomal abnormality. Even minor maternal disease, or such factors as the mother smoking during pregnancy, may profoundly affect the growth of the fetus, producing a "small for gestational age" baby.

Nevertheless, small and lighter mothers tend to have "smaller for dates" babies than tall or heavier mothers. Obese mothers tend to have fat babies. A recent study (Roberts and Powell, 1975) has revealed a strong interrelation between malformations. 84% of lung defects, 70% of kidney defects, 34% of eye defects, 19% of cleft palate and 15% of spina bifida coexisted with other defects; this has been taken as evidence against the notion that multiple external factors are involved in the causation of human malformations. Nowadays, it is possible to detect certain anomalies in a fetus by performing amniocentesis (see p. 35) and observing the cellular and chemical characteristics of the amniotic fluid which is withdrawn. Thus, the level of alpha-fetoprotein is increased in cases where the fetus has a defect of the neural tube (anencephaly or meningomyelocele), exomphalos, sacrococcygeal tumour, oesophageal or duodenal atresia, Fallot's tetrad and when intra-uterine death of the fetus occurs.

The gynaecologist must frequently examine an embryo which has been aborted and give an estimate of its age. This is possible by measuring the crown-rump length (C.R. length or sitting height) of the embryo and referring to tables (see, for example, Hamilton, Boyd and Mossman, 1972). By the end of the first month of development the C.R. length is 5 mm but this increases to 30 mm at the end of the second month. Streeter (1942, 1945, 1948) documented the features of embryos at various periods and described 23 age groups to indicate the levels of development (developmental horizons). Embryos of the first three weeks of development have recently been classified into nine stages (O'Rahilly, 1973).

From the beginning of the third month onwards, the developing human is called a fetus and it is mainly during this time that growth occurs, organs and tissues having already differentiated to a great extent in the embryonic period, during the first two months.

The textbook by Gray and Skandalakis (1972) should be consulted for a more extensive description of surgical anomalies. Details of incidence of anomalies in the following pages have been derived from that book.

References

Baer, K. E. von (1828). "Ueber Entwicklungsgeschichte der Thiere" Konigsberg.

Brachet, J. (1944). "Embryologie Chimique" Masson, Paris.

Brachet, J. (1967). The Living Cell *In* "Human Variations and Origins" Chap. 5, pp. 61-71. W. H. Freeman, San Francisco.

de Beer, Sir Gavin (1958). "Embryos and Ancestors" Clarendon Press, Oxford.

Gaillard, P. J. (1954). Greffes à l'homme de tissus cultivés *in vitro*. *Rev. méd. Liège* **9**, 271-276.

Geber, W. F. (1966). Developmental effects of chronic maternal audiovisual stress on the rat fetus. *J. Embryol. exp. Morph.* **16**, 1-16.

Giroud, A. and Lefebvres, J. (1957). Déficiences nutritionnelles tératogènes. *Ann. Nutrit. Aliment.* **11**, 15-49.

Gray, S. W. and Skandalakis, J. E. (1972). "Embryology for Surgeons" W. B. Saunders, London.

Hamilton, W. J., Boyd, J. D. and Mossman, H. W. (1972). "Human Embryology" (4th edn) Heffer, Cambridge.

Hieger, I. and Pullinger, B. D. (1953). *In* "Recent Advances in Pathology" (Ed. G. Hadfield, 6th edn) Chap. 5, p. 102. Churchill, London.

Jacobson, W. (1958). *In* "A Symposium on the Evaluation of Drug Toxicity" (Ed. A. Walpole and A. Spinks) pp. 76-103. Churchill, London.

Kalter, H. and Warkany, J. (1959). Experimental production of congenital malformations in mammals by metabolic procedure. *Physiol. Rev.* **39**, 69-115.

Lison, L. (1953). "Histochimie et Cytochimie Animales" (2nd edn) Gauthier-Villars, Paris.

Needham, J. (1931). "Chemical Embryology" (3 Vols) Camb. Univ. Press.

Needham, J. (1950). "Biochemistry and Morphogenesis" Camb. Univ. Press.

O'Rahilly, R. (1973). "Development stages in Human Embryos" Part A. Carnegie Institute of Washington.

Quastel, J. H. and Bickis, I. J. (1959). Metabolism of normal tissues and neoplasms in vitro. *Nature, Lond.* **183**, 281-286.

Rao, C. R. (1958). Some statistical methods for comparison of growth curves. *Biometrics* **14**, 1-17.

Raven, Chr. P. (1959). "An Outline of Developmental Physiology" Pergamon Press, Oxford.

Roberts, C. J. and Powell, R. G. (1975). Interrelation of the common congenital malformations. *Lancet* **ii**, 848-9.

Rous, Peyton (1959). Surmise and fact on the nature of cancer. *Nature, Lond.* **183**, 1357-61.

Sever, J. L. (1967). *In* "Advances in Teratology" Vol. 2, Chap. 4 Logos Press, London.

Streeter, G. L. (1942). Developmental horizons in human embryos: age group XI, 13-20 somites, and age group XII, 21-29 somites. *Contr. Embryol.* **30**, 211-245.

Streeter, G. L. (1945). Developmental horizons in human embryos: age group XIII, embryos 4 or 5 mm. long and age group XIV, indentation of lens vesicle. *Contr. Embryol.* **31**, 26-63.

Streeter, G. L. (1948). Developmental horizons in human embryos: age groups XV, XVI, XVII XVIII, being the third issue of a survey of the Carnegie Collection. *Contr. Embryol.* **32**, 133-203.

Tanner, J. M. (1962). "Growth at Adolescence" Blackwell, Oxford.

Thompson, D'Arcy W. (1948). "On Growth and Form" Camb. Univ. Press.

Toner, P. G. and Carr, K. E. (1968). "Cell Structure" E. & S. Livingstone, Edinburgh.

Wegmann, T. G. and Gilman, J. G. (1970). Chimerism for three genetic systems in tetraparental mice. *Dev. Biol.* **21**, 281-291.

Weiss, P. (1939). "Principles of Development" Henry Holt, New York.

Weiss, P. (1953). Some introductory remarks on the cellular basis of differentiation. *J. Embryol. exp. Morph.* **1**, 181-211.

Willis, R. A. (1958). "The Borderland of Embryology and Pathology" Butterworth, London.

Wislocki, G. B. and Dempsey, E. W. (1948). The chemical histology of the human placenta and decidua with reference to mucopolysaccharides, glycogen, lipids and acid phosphatase. *Am. J. Anat.* **83**, 1-42.

Woollam, D. H. M. (1967). "Advances in Teratology" Vols 1 and 2. Logos Press, London.

Woollam, D. H. M. and Millen, J. W. (1960). "Ciba Foundation Colloquium on Congenital Malformations" p. 158. Churchill, London.

2

Spermatogenesis

Development commences by the process of fertilization, the fusion of male and female gametes, the spermatozoon and the ovum respectively, to form a zygote. Any consideration of development must therefore properly include a knowledge of both the male and the female reproductive apparatus. The component structures of the male reproductive system are the primary sex organ or gonad, which is the *testis,* the accessory sex organs, which include such structures as the *epididymis* and *ductus deferens,* the external genitalia, and certain glands which are associated with them, for example, the *seminal vesicles,* the *prostate* and the bulbo-urethral glands. The secondary sexual characteristics include such features as the timbre of the voice and the distribution of pubic hair. The testis lies outside the abdominal cavity in the scrotum, which is a specialized sac of skin. In this way it differs from the female sex organ or gonad, the ovary, which is intraperitoneal. The result of this, as may be observed when examining the temperature control of the testis, is that the temperature inside the testis is lower than that in the abdominal cavity and that spermatogenesis (the formation of spermatozoa) proceeds best at this temperature.

In the testis spermatogenesis proceeds within the seminiferous tubules, which occupy the lobules of the testis. Once formed the spermatozoa are transported in fluid secreted by the seminiferous tubules to the rete testis by rhythmic contractions of the tubules. From the rete testis the spermatozoa pass into the duct of the epididymis via the ductuli efferentes and eventually reach the tail of the epididymis where they await ejaculation.

Spermatogenic cells

When the testes of different mammals are examined histologically, it is astonishing how little difference there is between them (Harrison, 1956). The seminiferous tubules of an elephant, for example, are approximately the same diameter as those of a mouse and the cellular elements within the tubules are very similar in size and appearance. If a histological section of a seminiferous tubule is examined under high magnification (Fig. 3), a membrane, the membrana propria, can be seen around the periphery of the seminiferous tubule. Outside this are the cells of the *interstitial tissue,* most important of which are the Leydig cells. Lying immediately inside the membrana propria are two main types of cell. One type is not directly concerned with the process of spermatogenesis; this is the cell which is called the *Sertoli cell,* a non-spermatogenic cell type. It is sometimes called a sustentacular cell because it is said to nourish some spermatogenic cells. The

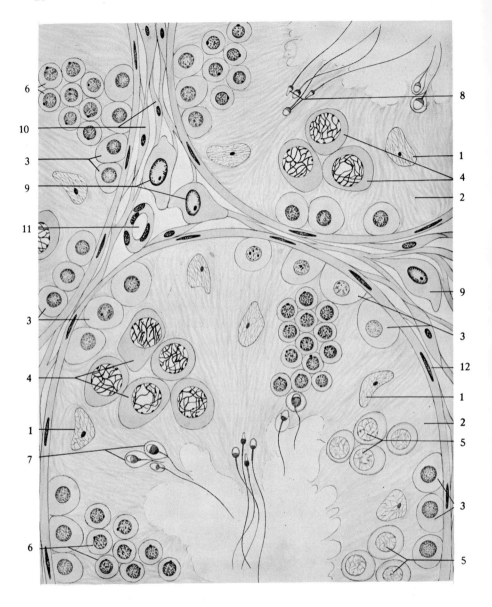

Fig. 3. Drawing of a histological section through parts of three human seminiferous tubules to show the cells involved in the various stages of spermatogenesis: 1 Nucleus of Sertoli cell; 2 Sertoli cell cytoplasm; 3 Spermatogonia; 4 Primary spermatocytes; 5 Secondary spermatocytes; 6 Spermatids; 7 Maturing spermatids with cytoplasmic droplets attached; 8 Spermatozoa; 9 Leydig cells; 10 Fibroblasts; 11 Blood vessel; 12 Membrana propria. Reproduced with permission of Oxford University Press from Cunningham's "Textbook of Anatomy", eleventh edition, 1972.

Sertoli cells also elaborate testicular fluid and maintain a blood-testis barrier (Fawcett, 1975). The other type of cell is of great importance in the process of spermatogenesis and is called a *spermatogonium*. By its division it produces cells which eventually divide again in order to form the mature spermatozoa. When it divides by mitosis it may either form two spermatogonia or two *primary spermatocytes*. The primary spermatocyte in turn divides to form two cells called *secondary spermatocytes* but the mechanism of this division is quite different and is called reduction division or *meiosis,* during which the number of chromosomes in the primary spermatocyte is exactly halved.

Disjunction of chromosomes

It is known that in the mature cells of the human being there are 46 chromosomes (Ford, Jacobs and Lajtha, 1958); this is termed the *diploid* number. Forty-four of these are exactly alike and are called autosomes but in the male two of them are unlike each other and unlike the other 44; they are called the X and Y chromosomes or sex chromosomes. 44XY is considered to be the chromosome constitution of the mature male cell. This is the chromosome constitution of the spermatogonium and also of the primary spermatocyte but when the primary spermatocyte divides and forms two secondary spermatocytes, then the number of chromosomes is halved to 23 (the *haploid* number) so that one secondary spermatocyte has 22X and the other 22Y chromosomes. This pattern of division ensures that at the time of fertilization the chromosome constitution of the spermatozoon will determine the sex of the offspring, which is in no way conditioned by the female germ cell, because the chromosome constitution of mature female cells is 44XX and each *secondary oocyte* resulting from the meiotic division of a *primary oocyte* has a chromosome constitution of 22X chromosomes. When a secondary oocyte is fertilized by a 22X spermatozoon, a female results but fertilization from a 22Y spermatozoon produces a male. Because of this difference in the chromosomes of the two sexes, variations occur in the appearance of the nuclei of mature *somatic* cells (Barr, Bertram and Lindsay, 1950). Since the nucleus of the adult female cell has a larger amount of sex chromatin, the female nucleus has a hemispherical chromatin body (the Barr body or "sex chromatin") about 1 mμ in diameter pressed against the nuclear membrane in approximately 70% of cells. During meiotic division of the primary spermatocyte or primary oocyte, each chromosome does not split as in mitosis. The chromosomes first come to lie beside one another in pairs and then the members of each pair separate—the so-called *disjunction* of chromosomes—into the two daughter cells. Consequently, each resultant secondary spermatocyte (and the spermatozoon which forms from it) or secondary oocyte normally contains 22 autosomes and one sex chromosome.

When the secondary spermatocyte divides, it does so by mitosis, although paradoxically this division is called the second maturation or second reduction division. The cells resulting from this division are called spermatids, which therefore have exactly the same chromosome constitution as the secondary spermatocytes. There is then no further division during spermatogenesis and the spermatids merely mature in order to form the adult spermatozoa. This maturation of the spermatids to form spermatozoa is called *spermiogenesis* or spermateliosis and the period of spermatogenesis up to the formation of spermatids is called *spermatocytogenesis*. Late spermatids can be easily recognized inside the seminiferous tubule because they have a granule applied to one side of the nucleus called the acrosome granule. This granule by eventual growth caps the nucleus and forms part of the head of the resultant spermatozoon. The spermatids as they are maturing attach themselves to the cytoplasm of the Sertoli cell and remain attached during spermiogenesis. During the period of attachment, they are very probably nourished by glucose or fructose formed by the breakdown of polysaccharides in the cytoplasm of the Sertoli cells.

The spermatozoa

The mature human spermatozoon (sperm) is a highly specialized cell, modified for the motility it needs to reach the ovum during fertilization (Fig. 4). It consists of a *head* (composed mostly of the nucleus) the shape of a flattened ellipsoid and capped by the acrosome, of mean length 4·4 mμ (van Duijn, 1958), a *middle piece,* approximately 5 mμ long, which consists mainly of a paired spiral thread probably formed from mitochondria and a *tail* 40-50 mμ in length which consists of two central filaments and nine pairs of circumferential filaments (Fawcett (1954) has shown that this number is also constant for all cilia examined) which are responsible for the movements of the tail and therefore the motility of the spermatozoon; these are surrounded by a tail sheath and are related anteriorly to the centriole, which is in the middle piece and lies just behind the head. The mature spermatozoon possesses little or no cytoplasm of the spermatid which gave origin to it; this is lost during spermiogenesis.

The semen ejaculated at coitus consists of the spermatozoa suspended in seminal plasma, which is secreted by the accessory organs of reproduction. The volume of semen in a single ejaculate and the sperm density per μlitre varies considerably amongst mammals (Mann, 1954), as can be seen from Table I; the volume of a single ejaculate in man also varies from 2 to 6 ml, and the sperm density from 50 to 150 million per ml. Approximately 20% of the spermatozoa in normal semen are abnormal in having, for example, small heads, pear-shaped or double heads, bifid tails (see Harvey and Jackson, 1945).

In addition to producing spermatozoa the testis is an endocrine gland and its Leydig cells are capable of secreting androgenic hormone, mostly in the form of the steroid hormone *testosterone.* This hormone is responsible for the integrity and growth of the accessory organs of reproduction and the

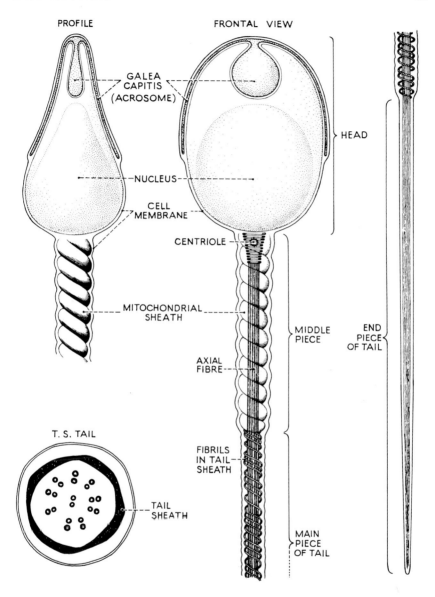

PROFILE

FRONTAL VIEW

GALEA
CAPITIS
(ACROSOME)

NUCLEUS

CELL
MEMBRANE

CENTRIOLE

HEAD

MIDDLE
PIECE

END
PIECE
OF TAIL

MITOCHONDRIAL
SHEATH

AXIAL
FIBRE

T. S. TAIL

FIBRILS
IN TAIL
SHEATH

TAIL
SHEATH

MAIN
PIECE
OF TAIL

Fig. 4. Diagrammatic representation of the appearance of a human spermatozoon as shown by electron microscopy. In frontal view the head of the spermatozoon is oval in shape but at right angles to this plane the head is piriform in shape. The spermatozoon is shown in two parts for ease of portrayal. When a transverse section is taken of the middle piece of the spermatozoon (bottom left of figure), it is seen to be composed of one central pair of filaments surrounded by nine additional pairs, all being enclosed in a sheath. The filaments constitute the axial fibre, which continues into the tail and is responsible for its movements.

Table I. Species Differences in Volume and Sperm Density of Ejaculated Semen

| Species | Volume of single ejaculate | | Sperm density in semen | |
	Normal variations (ml)	Most common value (ml)	Normal variations (sperm/μl)	Average value (sperm/μl)
Ass	10-80	50	200,000-600,000	400,000
Bat		0·05	5,000,000-8,000,000	6,000,000
Boar	150-500	250	25,000-300,000	100,000
Bull	2-10	4	300,000-2,000,000	1,000,000
Cock	0·2-1·5	0·8	50,000-6,000,000	3,500,000
Dog	2-15	6	1,000,000-9,000,000	3,000,000
Fox	0·2-4	1·5	30,000-250,000	70,000
Man	2-6	3·5	50,000-150,000	100,000
Rabbit	0·4-6	1	100,000-2,000,000	700,000
Ram	0·7-2	1	2,000,000-5,000,000	3,000,000
Stallion	30-300	70	30,000-800,000	120,000
Turkey	0·2-0·8	0·3		7,000,000

presence of secondary sexual characteristics. It also has an anabolic effect on body proteins and is related to body growth, since orchidectomy (i.e. castration, the removal of the testes) prepubertally causes an increase in height due to delayed ossification of the epiphysial cartilages. The testis in turn is under the control of hormones secreted by the anterior lobe of the pituitary gland; *follicle stimulating hormone* (F.S.H.) stimulates the growth of the Graafian follicle in the ovary (see p. 18) and is identical with a hormone in the male which stimulates spermatogenesis, while *interstitial-cell stimulating hormone* (I.C.S.H.), which is identical with the female luteinizing hormone, stimulates the growth and development of interstitial tissue.

CLINICAL RELATIONSHIPS

Abnormally, disjunction of chromosomes may fail to occur during meiosis and affects the sex chromosomes most commonly. Such non-disjunction of sex chromosomes can result in spermatozoa with 22XY chromosomes or 22 autosomes and in secondary oocytes with 22XX chromosomes or 22 autosomes. Germ cells with such an abnormal chromosome constitution are able to participate in fertilization, so that offspring are known with a chromosomé constitution 44XXY (Klinefelter's syndrome), 44X (Turner's syndrome), or even 44XXX (the "super female" or triple X female). Such syndromes are seldom transmitted and their overall frequency is about 5 per 1000 live births. Men with *Klinefelter's syndrome* possess male external genitalia, but the penis is often small and the testes small and firm. Spermatogenesis is completely or almost entirely absent and the seminiferous tubules may contain only Sertoli cells. The bodily habitus varies; some are normal in size, others tall and eunuchoid, or there may be a feminine distribution of body fat, a smooth skin and a general absence of body and pubic hair. Some men may have gynaecomastia (enlargement of the breasts). Mental retardation is common.

Individuals with *Turner's syndrome* may present as men or women with characteristic webbing of the neck, a short stature and testicular or ovarian dysgenesis; the secondary sexual characteristics are poorly developed and there may be a narrowing (stenosis) of the aorta. The webbed neck consists of folds of skin extending from the ear to the shoulder, which do not involve the trapezius muscle. X-radiography may reveal rarefaction of bones and a deformity of the thorax, such as "shield-like chest" or "pigeon chest" may occur. The *super female* may have a normal physical habitus and may be tall with good muscular development; there may be mental retardation and disturbance of menstruation. The defect in this condition is one form of *trisomy,* in contrast to the *monosomy* of Turner's syndrome.

Non-disjunction may also affect autosomes, leading to monosomy or trisomy. Such defects are usually incompatible with normal development and the embryos abort. The majority of patients with *Down's syndrome,* however, have been shown to be trisomic for the autosome labelled as chromosome 21. The incidence of this syndrome is placed as high as 1 in 600 births and all available evidence favours non-disjunction during maternal oogenesis as the factor resulting in the birth of such a child. The frequency rises with increasing maternal age (5% for mothers over the age of 38). Because children with this syndrome have slanted eyes and an epicanthic skin fold, the condition used to be termed *mongolism.* The mongol child is an idiot or mentally retarded and has characteristic dermatoglyphics. Growth may be retarded.

Factors affecting spermatogenesis

Many factors are known to influence spermatogenesis (Harrison, 1956) but the testis shows a uniform histological response to damaging influences, suggesting that some final common factor such as ischaemia or anoxia, may be responsible. Ischaemia (a deficiency of blood) in itself, effected by interference with the flow of blood through the testicular artery, produces profound changes which may lead to complete destruction of all spermatogenic cells in the tubules or even destruction of Sertoli cells in addition, depending on the severity of the ischaemia. Obstruction of the ductuli efferentes (see Harrison, 1956), interruption of the epididymal arteries (Macmillan, 1953), an environmental temperature above 40°C *locally applied* to the scrotum (see Moore, 1939; Harrison, 1975) or below 8°C (Macdonald and Harrison, 1954) applied to the scrotum, hypophysectomy (removal of the pituitary gland), large doses of female sex hormone (oestrogenic hormone) or even of androgenic hormone (see Harrison, 1958), can also lead to the same degenerative changes. Environmental temperature is rather important and it has been suggested that the reason for lack of spermatogenesis in the undescended (cryptorchid) testis is the fact that it is at a higher temperature than it would normally be subjected to in the scrotum. The mechanism of maintenance of the testis at its normal temperature inside the scrotum depends on several factors; thus it has been shown that the variation in abdomino-testicular temperature difference in mammals depends on the degree of convolution of the testicular artery (Harrison and Weiner, 1949). Among other factors which must also be considered are the intrinsic heat production of the testis and the character of the scrotal skin. It is understandable that any mechanism preventing loss of heat from the scrotum will also affect spermatogenesis adversely; the character of a man's underclothing and the frequency and temperature of his bath may therefore be factors of importance to his fertility. One of the first effects on spermatogenesis of these adverse factors is an interference with spermiogenesis; since the spermatids cannot mature they produce *multinucleate* cells. As the testicular artery is surrounded by the veins of the pampiniform plexus, heat transfer can occur between them so enabling thermo-regulatory control of testicular temperature. In *varicocele,* a varicose condition of the cremasteric veins or the veins of the pampiniform plexus, this mechanism is upset and spermatogenic tissue degenerates. Although usually occurring unilaterally, spermatogenic damage is frequently found in the contralateral testis. This is probably due to the fact that the degenerating spermatogenic tissue acts as an auto-antigen inducing an immune reaction in the other testis which results in spermatogenic damage there. All of the phenomena outlined above are of great importance in the diagnosis and treatment of human infertility and sterility and this has been treated more completely elsewhere (Harrison and de Boer, 1976).

In congenital absence of the ductus deferens, spermatozoa are completely absent from the semen, a condition called azoospermia. In oligospermia the ejaculate volume is less than 0.5 ml and the density of spermatozoa less than 30 million per ml. The seminal plasma contains many substances (see Mann, 1954) such as citric acid, fructose, phosphorylcholine, inositol and the organic compounds spermine and spermidine which are responsible for the characteristic odour of semen; the spermine can crystallize out from semen as a phosphate to form "Boettcher's crystals", and is the substance responsible for Barberio's reaction used in forensic medicine for the chemical detection of human semen. The mammalian testis and the spermatozoa themselves are the richest known animal source of the enzyme hyaluronidase, which brings about depolymerization and hydrolysis of hyaluronic acid. It has been suggested that this hyaluronidase enables the spermatozoon to enter the ovum at fertilization and Austin (1961) claims that the function of the acrosome is most likely to be the carriage of hyaluronidase, which enables the spermatozoon to pass through the cumulus oophorus, the matrix of which is rich in hyaluronic acid. Some authors regard the acrosome as a large lysosome (see Fig. 4).

References

Austin, C. R. (1961). "The Mammalian Egg" Blackwell Scientific Publications, Oxford.

Barr, M. L., Bertram, L. F. and Lindsay, H. A. (1950). The morphology of the nerve cell nucleus, according to sex. *Anat. Rec.* **107**, 283-298.

Duijn, C. Van, Jnr. (1958). Biometry of human spermatozoa. *Jl R. Microsc. Soc.* **77**, 12-27.

Fawcett, D. W. (1954). The study of epithelial cilia and sperm flagella with the electron microscope. *The Laryngoscope* **64**, 557-567.

Fawcett, D. W. (1975). Ultrastructure and function of the Sertoli cell. *Handbook of Physiology*, Section 7, Vol. 5, Chap. 2, pp. 21-55.

Ford, C. E., Jacobs, P. A. and Lajtha, L. G. (1958). Human somatic chromosomes. *Nature, Lond.* **181**, 1565-68.

Harrison, R. G. (1956). Factors influencing the process of spermatogenesis in the experimental animal. *Br. J. Urol.* **28**, 422-5.

Harrison, R. G. (1958). Facteurs vasculaires dans la physiologie normale de la spermatogénèse. *In* "La Fonction Spermatogénétique du Testicule" pp. 63-72. Masson, Paris.

Harrison, R. G. (1975). Effect of temperature on the mammalian testis *In* "Handbook of Physiology" Section 7, Vol. 5, Chap. 9, pp. 219-223.

Harrison, R. G. and de Boer, C. (1976). "Sex and Infertility" Academic Press, London.

Harrison, R. G. and Weiner, J. S. (1949). Vascular patterns of the mammalian testis and their functional significance. *J. exp. Biol.* **26**, 304-316.

Harvey, C. and Jackson, M. H. (1945). Assessment of male fertility by semen analysis. *Lancet* **249**, 99-104.

Macdonald, J. and Harrison, R. G. (1954). Effect of low temperatures on rat spermatogenesis. *Fertil. Steril.* **5**, 205-216.

Macmillan, E. W. (1953). Higher epididymal obstructions in male infertility. *Fertil. Steril.* **4**, 101-127.

Mann, T. (1954). "The Biochemistry of Semen" Methuen, London.

Moore, C. R. (1939). *In* "Sex and Internal Secretions" (Ed. E. Allen) Chap. 7, p. 353. Bailliere, Tindall and Cox, London.

3

Oogenesis

In the female the primary sex organ or gonad is the *ovary*. The position of the human ovary differs from that of the testis in that it lies inside the abdominal cavity in a fossa on the lateral wall of the pelvis called the ovarian fossa. Because it develops in exactly the same situation as the testis, that is, in the region corresponding to the position of the kidney in adult life, it must also descend to a certain extent during development. For a similar reason the ovarian arteries arise from the abdominal aorta near the renal artery; the ovarian vein also drains into the inferior vena cava on the right side and on the left into the left renal vein. The accessory reproductive organs in the female comprise the *uterus* or *womb,* the *uterine (Fallopian) tubes,* the *vagina, external genitalia* and *mammary glands.* The secondary sexual characteristics include such features as the characteristic distribution of subcutaneous fat, timbre of the voice and distribution of pubic hair.

Just as in the male, the female accessory reproductive organs depend for their integrity on secretions produced by the ovary. If both ovaries are removed, the accessory reproductive organs regress.

Oogenesis, the production of ova, occurs in the cortex of the ovary. At the time of birth, the ovary contains all the potential germ cells that are likely to mature into ova during the life span of a woman (see Zuckerman, 1951). This pool of about a million primary oocytes has already been formed from other mother cells (the oogonia) during prenatal life. By the time of puberty, this number has been considerably reduced and about 40,000 primary oocytes remain. Each primary oocyte is to be found within an ovarian follicle, where it is surrounded by follicular cells. During each menstrual cycle after puberty, a small group of follicles attempt to mature; only one usually succeeds in doing so; the others degenerate and become *atretic*. In the successful follicle, blocks of homogeneous material develop in between the primary oocyte and the follicular cells and these later become confluent to form a membrane called the *zona pellucida*. The follicular cells then begin to proliferate and increase greatly in number to form the "granulosa cells" (Fig. 5). A cavity then appears amongst the granulosa cells and this enlarges so much that the oocyte is pushed out to the periphery of the follicle (Fig. 6), which, when fully formed, is termed a *Graafian follicle,* since Regnier de Graaf (1677) first described it. When fully formed, this follicle is a prominent structure and can be seen on the surface of the ovary by the naked eye. A collection of the granulosa cells called the *cumulus oophorus* surrounds the oocyte at the periphery of the follicle. The ovarian stroma surrounding the

18

follicle forms a *theca interna* (or thecal gland, because it is thought to secrete one type of female sex hormone called oestrogenic hormone). Immediately outside the theca interna there is another layer of cells called the *theca externa* which forms a fibrous capsule. Finally, the primary oocyte undergoes the first reduction division to form a secondary oocyte; the second reduction division commences and the Graafian follicle liberates the secondary oocyte

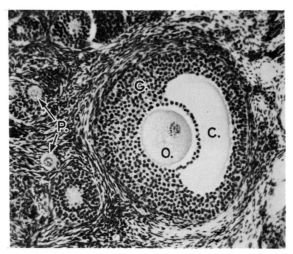

Fig. 5. A developing Graafian follicle from the ovary of a macaque monkey. The follicle contains an oocyte (O.) and granulosa cells (G.) in which a cavity (C.) has just appeared. Some primordial follicles (P.) are also present. ($\times$ 132).

into the uterine tube. The distension of the follicle and its eventual breakdown at the surface of the ovary is associated with a dissociation and reduction in number of collagen fibres in the wall of the follicle, accomplished by an "ovulatory enzyme" with properties similar to collagenase (Rondell, 1970). If fertilization occurs, the second reduction division is completed. The ruptured and collapsed Graafian follicle becomes transformed, in the post-ovulatory period, into a *corpus luteum,* by an enlargement and proliferation of the granulosa cells, which become filled with lipid. This then becomes fibrosed as a *corpus albicans.* The corpus luteum secretes another hormone, called *progesterone.*

Menstrual cycle

The length of the menstrual cycle, a periodic phenomenon related to ovulation, is, on average, 28 days. The first day of the menstrual flow is considered as the beginning of the menstrual cycle and the cycle ends at the 28th day, which is the day preceding the first day of the next menstrual flow. Ovulation occurs 14 ± 3 days before the next expected menstrual flow, and therefore in a 28-day cycle occurs in the middle of the menstrual cycle.

The pre-ovulatory phase of the menstrual cycle is also termed the follicular phase and the post-ovulatory phase the luteal phase. Because the hormones secreted by the ovary affect the accessory reproductive organs, there are marked changes in the endometrium (the mucous membrane of the uterus) coincident with the changes occurring in the ovary. Thus, during the follicular phase of the menstrual cycle, under the influence of oestrogenic

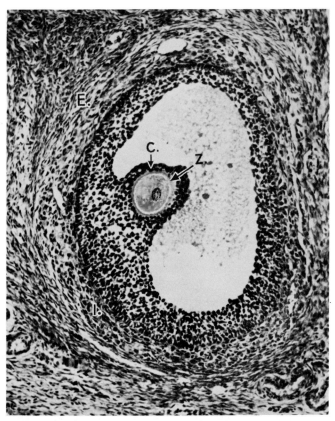

Fig. 6. A human Graafian follicle in which the follicular cavity has enlarged to such an extent that a cumulus oophorus (C.) has formed. The oocyte is surrounded by a zona pellucida (Z.). The follicle is surrounded by a theca interna (I.) and theca externa (E.). ($\times$ 180).

hormones, there is proliferation of the endometrium, while during the luteal phase of the cycle, progesterone causes secretory changes to occur; the histological appearances of the *proliferative* and *secretory* types of endometrium are depicted in Figs 7 and 8.

The endometrium is composed of a *stratum compactum* containing the necks of the uterine glands, the *stratum spongiosum,* which contains the bodies of the glands, and the *stratum basalis* containing the bases of the glands (Fig. 8). The stratum basalis has its own blood supply and is never shed but the other two superficial layers, which are supplied by longer arteries which become coiled in the secretory phase, disintegrate to produce the menstrual flow. The two types of artery have been described by Daron (1936) and Bartelmez (1957).

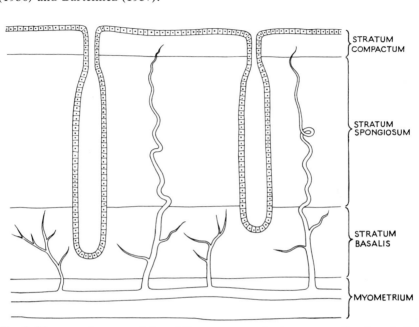

Fig. 7. Diagrammatic representation of the appearance of a transverse section through the endometrium in the pre-ovulatory (proliferative) phase.

The epithelium of the endometrium dips down at intervals into the subjacent stroma in order to form tubular glands. These glands are quite simple in the proliferative phase but in the post-ovulatory period they become increasingly corkscrew in outline in histological section. The endometrium thickens considerably in the proliferative phase; in the secretory phase there is no further thickening but the glands become tortuous, as also do the arteries within the endometrium. This change is preparatory for the implantation (nidation or imbedding) of the blastocyst, should fertilization occur. The secretory changes occurring in the endometrium are also preparatory for the arrival of the dividing fertilized ovum in the uterine lumen, for there is a free "floating" period which it spends in the uterine cavity before implantation. If fertilization does not occur, the stratum compactum and stratum spongiosum of the endometrium disintegrate and form the menstrual flow, leaving the stratum basalis with its own independent blood supply to regenerate the endometrium in the next succeeding menstrual cycle.

There is a reciprocal relationship between the pituitary gland and the secretion of hormones by the ovary. The anterior lobe of the pituitary gland controls the other endocrine glands in the body by producing secretions which influence their activity. Two of these are of importance for the gonads. They are called follicle stimulating hormone (F.S.H.) and luteinizing hormone (L.H.), whose names describe their action exactly. F.S.H. stimulates growth of the ovarian follicle, while L.H. stimulates the growth of the corpus luteum.

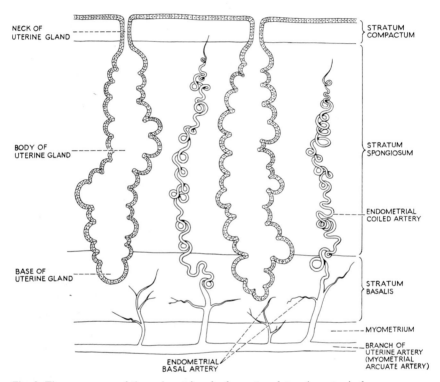

Fig. 8. The appearance of the endometrium in the post-ovulatory (secretory) phase.

As the ovarian follicle grows the amount of oestrogenic hormone secreted by the theca interna increases, reaches a maximum at the time of ovulation and then begins to fall until the onset of the next menstrual cycle. Because the corpus luteum forms immediately after ovulation, progesterone is not secreted by the ovary until after ovulation, and since the corpus luteum begins to regress a few days before the next expected menstrual flow, the secretion of progesterone therefore decreases at that time. At the beginning of the menstrual cycle the theca interna is relatively poorly developed and therefore the amount of oestrogenic hormone secreted by it is small. Such small amounts of oestrogenic hormone circulating in the blood stimulate a further increase in F.S.H. production. When the secretion of oestrogenic hormone exceeds a certain threshold level, however, the converse applies; it suppresses the secretion of F.S.H. and the pituitary then commences to secrete L.H., which in turn causes the transformation of the ruptured Graafian follicle into a corpus luteum. Similar hormonal relationships then apply. Small amounts of progesterone secreted by this corpus luteum stimulate further secretion of L.H., but when the secretion of progesterone rises above a certain threshold level, L.H. secretion is depressed. The same sort of reciprocal relation with the pituitary applies to the testis and the secretion of testosterone, the cortex of the suprarenal gland, the thyroid gland and possibly other endocrine glands in the body. This depression of the gonadotrophic activity of the pituitary by oestrogenic and progestational hormones and, therefore, consequent suppression of ovulation, is the basis of the action of the contraceptive pill, although other factors, such as a change in viscosity of uterine cervical mucus, are involved. The secretion of gonadotrophic hormones is under the control of a gonadotrophin-releasing hormone, secreted by the hypothalamus.

Menstruation

The menstrual flow was claimed by Hartman, Firor and Geiling (1930) to be caused by a positive "bleeding" factor, secreted by the anterior lobe of the pituitary. It was later shown by Zuckerman (1936) and many others that this is untrue. Macaque monkeys in which both ovaries had been removed were injected with oestrogenic hormone. When this was done it was found that the endometrium of the uteri of the monkeys could be maintained in a healthy condition; provided the level of oestrogenic hormone was kept above a certain threshold level, the endometrium remained in a proliferative state. If injections of oestrogenic hormone were then stopped suddenly, menstruation occurred. In other words, menstruation can be caused by the withdrawal of oestrogenic hormone at least. To other monkeys in which both of the ovaries had been removed, Zuckerman later administered oestrogenic hormone and also injections of progesterone. It was found that a phase of luteal activity may be superimposed on a threshold level of oestrogenic hormone without affecting the periodicity of the bleeding. Other observations (see Hoffman, 1944) have shown that adequate amounts of progesterone can delay the onset of the menstrual flow but that normal menstruation can occur in the presence of large quantities of oestrogenic hormone. It may be concluded that the menstrual flow is a negative phenomenon occasioned by the withdrawal of both oestrogenic hormones and progesterone.

When fertilization occurs, however, there is no further menstrual flow, because the level of progesterone is maintained above the threshold level, since the corpus luteum of menstruation becomes transformed into a corpus luteum of pregnancy which is a very much larger and more persistent structure. Therefore, *amenorrhoea,* or the absence of menstrual flow, is one of the cardinal signs of pregnancy. That does not mean to say, however, that amenorrhoea invariably occurs, because very rarely there are cases in which there is a very slight menstrual flow after pregnancy has commenced. When the endometrium is acted upon by progesterone in pregnancy, it increases in its complexity. It becomes more vascular and the secretory character of the glands becomes even more marked. The stroma or connective tissue of the endometrium also changes in character; the cells of which it is composed become larger and paler, the so-called decidual cells and the endometrium is now called *decidua.*

It has been shown that cyclical changes occur in the epithelium of the uterine tubes, cellular content of the vagina and the rheological properties of a plug of mucus in the canal of the cervix uteri coincident with changes in the endometrium. Indeed the whole of the accessory reproductive apparatus is dependent on the hormonal relationships of the ovary and cyclical changes occur in it coincidentally with the changes proceeding in the ovary, which in turn is under the influence of the anterior lobe of the pituitary gland.

It is important that the process of ovulation and the factors which influence it should be considered in greater detail. First of all the terms should be defined. The word "puberty" is loosely used to indicate the time in an individual's life when maturation changes are occurring and he or she is becoming adult. It is not a very specific term, however, and therefore other words are necessary. Thus *menarche* is used to describe the time of onset of menstrual flows. Ashley Montagu (1946) has pointed out that ovulation does not necessarily commence at the menarche. The onset of ovulation he terms *nubility,* in other words the capacity of the female viably to conceive and reproduce. Since menarche and the time of nubility do not coincide there may be a period of anything from one month to seven years between the menarche and nubility. In that period obviously a woman will be sterile, because although she is menstruating, she is not ovulating, and therefore it has been termed the adolescent-sterility interval.

CLINICAL RELATIONSHIPS

A woman who never ovulates is sterile. It is therefore essential to be aware of the factors which can affect ovulation and of the methods whereby the gynaecologist can determine whether ovulation is occurring normally in the investigation of an infertile or sterile woman.

A condition of prolonged and excessive secretion of oestrogens with relatively poor secretion of progesterone, which is known to occur abnormally in some women, produces endometrial hyperplasia; in this disease ovulation does not usually occur. Since the rabbit will only ovulate following coitus and the ferret in response to light, it is obvious that ovulation is also governed by the activity of the nervous system, which is probably effected through the hypothalamus and the release of gonado-trophins.

Ovulation does not occur after the onset of pregnancy, though in rare cases it may do so and fertilization of this ovum might take place—the phenomenon of *superfetation*. In other words, the woman eventually gives birth to two children from two different conceptions, but born at the same time. The *puerperium* is the period immediately after parturition or birth, in which there may be ovulation without menstruation, although a woman who continues to suckle her child may not ovulate. Pathological changes, alterations in the blood supply of the uterus and other endocrine disorders can also affect ovulation. It is possible to study the cyclical changes in the accessory reproductive organs in the human being by endometrial biopsy, the removal of a small piece of endometrium to examine it histologically, by means of a small biopsy curette. Examination of this endometrium histologically in the post-ovulatory period demonstrates the presence or absence of secretory changes. In some women there is a small menstrual flow, the *Kleine Regel,* at the time of ovulation and in others a pain in one or other iliac fossa, the *Mittelschmerz* (see Krohn, 1954), possibly caused by the oocyte being liberated from the surface of the ovary. Changes in the *basal body temperature* also occur in the menstrual cycle (Harrison and de Boer, 1976). During the pre-ovulatory phase of the menstrual cycle, this temperature is lower than that following ovulation. Bailey and Marshall (1970) have shown that the post-ovulatory hyperthermic phase increases in length in a rectilinear fashion from 10 to 13 days as the total cycle length rises from 22 to 29 days: over total cycle lengths from 29 to 33 days the length of the hyperthermic phase stays around 13 days.

References

Bailey, J. and Marshall, J. (1970). The relationship of the post-ovulatory phase of the menstrual cycle to total cycle length. *J. biosoc. Sci.* **2,** 123-132.

Bartelmez, G. W. (1957). The form and functions of the uterine blood vessels in the rhesus monkey. *Contr. Embryol.* **36,** 153-182.

Daron, G. H. (1936). The arterial pattern of the tunica mucosa of the uterus in Macacus rhesus. *Am. J. Anat.* **58,** 349-419.

Graaf, Regnier de (1677). "Opera Omnia" Lugd. Batav.

Harrison, R. G. and de Boer, C. (1976). "Sex and Infertility" Academic Press, London.

Hartman, C. G., Firor, W. M. and Geiling, E. M. K. (1930). The anterior lobe and menstruation. *Am. J. Physiol.* **95,** 662-669.

Hoffman, J. (1944). "Female Endocrinology" Saunders, London.

Krohn, P. L. (1954). Clinical intermenstrual pain: the mittelschmerz. *J. Clin. Endocr.* **14,** 682-684.

Montagu, M. F. A. (1946). "Adolescent Sterility" Chas. C. Thomas, Springfield.

Rondell, P. (1970). Biophysical aspects of ovulation. *Biol. Reprod.* Supp. 2: 64-88.

Zuckerman, S. (1936). The nature of the oestrin-stimulus in uterine bleeding. *J. Physiol.* **87,** 51P-53P.

Zuckerman, S. (1951). The number of oocytes in the mature ovary. *Recent. Prog. Horm. Res.* **6,** 63-109.

4

Fertilization and the Formation of the Blastocyst

It has been estimated that the weight of an ovum is 15 ten-millionths of a gramme. The weight of a full term mature fetus is on average 3250 grammes. During the process of development there is therefore an increase in weight of approximately 2 billion times (Corner, 1944). Fertilization, the union of sperm and ovum, initiates this process and stimulates the occurrence of *cleavage,* or division of the fertilized ovum. But there are many other phenomena which occur at the time of fertilization (Rothschild, 1956; Austin and Bishop, 1957). One of the first consequences is *activation,* a name that has been applied to the detailed changes which occur in the structure and chemistry of the fertilized ovum. For example, it has been shown that there is a decrease in solubility and an increase in viscosity of egg proteins, a change of electrical conductivity and an increase of respiratory activity. Secondly there is a restoration of the diploid number of chromosomes by the fusion of two germ cells each containing a haploid number. The sex of the resultant individual is also determined at fertilization by the type of spermatozoon that fertilizes the ovum, i.e. depending on whether it is an X or Y spermatozoon, a female or a male is produced respectively. The chromosomes from each gamete also contribute their own genetic factors. Only when fertilization occurs and the spermatozoon penetrates the ovum is the second reduction division completed. In other words, only at that time is the mature ovum formed and the second polar body shed into the perivitelline space (Fig. 9), the first polar body having already been produced in the first reduction division (a meiotic division), inside the ovary. When reduction division occurs in spermatogenesis two cells which are more or less alike are usually formed but in oogenesis reduction division results in the formation of one large cell, which will develop into the mature ovum, and also a rather small structure, a *polar body,* the nature of which is obscure, apart from the fact that it constitutes a mechanism by which the total egg mass ejects half of its chromosomes and conserves a single ovum. After the spermatozoon penetrates the oocyte its head forms a male *pronucleus;* this fuses with the female pronucleus to form the *zygote,* which then starts to divide.

Development on the blastocyst

In the process of division or *cleavage* at first two cells are formed (Fig. 10). Of these two cells one is larger than the other and this then divides, so that only three cells are present after the second division. Then the other cell divides,

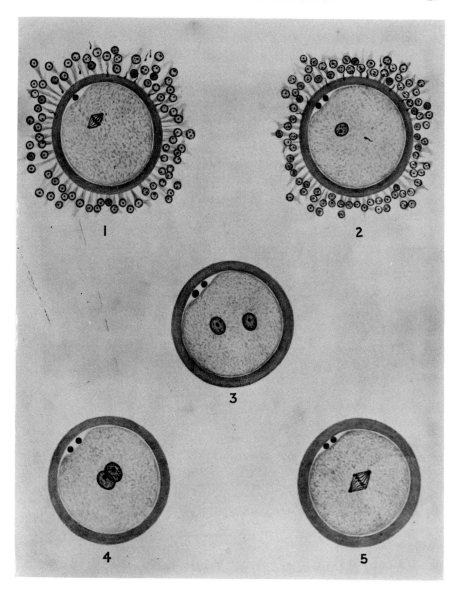

Fig. 9. The process of maturation of the oocyte and fertilization. In 1 the secondary oocyte, shed from the Graafian follicle, and surrounded by its zona pellucida and corona radiata (adherent cumulus oophorus cells), has its second maturation spindle. The first polar body is in the perivitelline space and the second reduction division is occuring. In 2 a sperm has penetrated into the cytoplasm of the ovum, and the second polar body has formed. In 3 the sperm has formed the male pronucleus; in 4 the two pronuclei are approximating, and in 5, cleavage is commencing.

so producing four cells and so on (Fig. 10), so that there is a linear increase in the number of cells. As cleavage is progressing the zygote passes down the uterine tube and when the process has reached the stage of producing 12-16 cells, the dividing zygote is called a *morula* and at this stage it appears in the uterine cavity. During the process of cleavage there is a synthesis of nuclear proteins from RNA in order to maintain the proper relationship between the amount of nuclear and cytoplasmic material. The cellular processes whereby

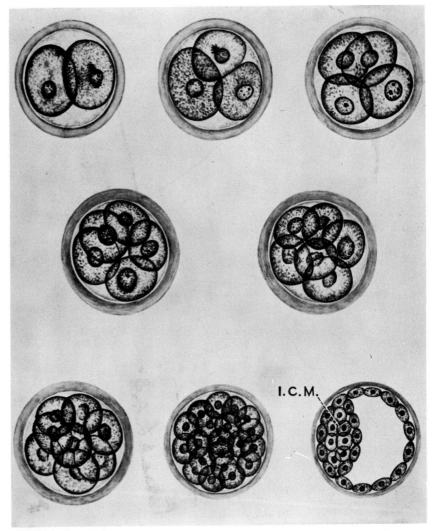

Fig. 10. The process of cleavage which produces a morula; a cavity (the blastocele) appears in this separating overlying trophoblast cells from the inner cell mass (I.C.M.) in the resultant spherical blastocyst.

this protein synthesis is effected are similar to those which occur in mitosis and cell regeneration and are outlined on p. 240. Since Hertig *et al.* (1954) recovered a 12-cell morula aged 3 days from the uterine cavity and a two-cell stage age 1½-2½ days has been isolated (Hertig and Rock, 1951) from the uterine tube (Fig. 11), the exact time relations of this process are more

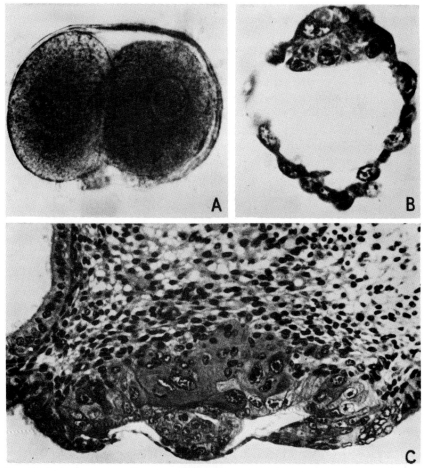

Fig. 11. A. An intact two-cell segmenting human egg, with the upper and smaller of the two polar bodies visible between the two blastomeres. Carnegie 8698, section 12. (× 500).
B. A mid-section through a 107 cell human blastocyst of which 8 are large vacuolated formative (embryonic) cells (the inner cell mass, seen at the top of the figure), and 99 are trophoblastic cells. Carnegie 8663, section 9. (× 600).
C. A recently implanted human ovum, not more than 7½ days of age. There is a concentration of dark syncytiotrophoblast in the centre of the implantation site dorsal to the embryo (seen at the middle of the bottom of the figure). The lighter cytotrophoblast is most prominent peripherally, but also lines the inner surface of the proliferating trophoblast dorsal to the embryo, and is amniogenic at its area of contact with the embryo. The embryonic disc is bilaminar and an amniotic cavity is present. Below the endoderm is a layer of unchanged, flattened trophoblastic cells, one cell thick. Carnegie 8020, section 6-5-9. (× 300).

completely understood. In addition, by extrapolation from the findings in an investigation of the process of cleavage in the macaque monkey (Heuser and Streeter, 1941), it may be presumed that the human morula appears in the uterine cavity on or about the third day after fertilization; it remains in the uterine cavity in the fluid secreted by the uterine glands. It will be remembered that in the immediate post-ovulatory phase secretory changes occur in the glands of the endometrium; when fertilization takes place these become more pronounced in the decidua which has the capacity of secreting larger quantities of fluid from its glands. This fluid passes into the morula in between its various cells to form a cavity. When this happens, the morula is termed a *blastocyst* and the cavity in the blastocyst, filled with fluid, is called the segmentation cavity. Free human blastocysts, aged 4-4½ days, have been isolated from the uterine cavity (see Fig. 11 and Hertig, Rock and Adams, 1956). The blastocyst is spherical and is composed of an outer shell of cells immediately underneath the zona pellucida called the *trophoblast,* while at one pole of the blastocyst there is a small clump of cells called the *inner cell mass,* which is itself covered by trophoblast (Figs 10, 11). All of the changes which produce a blastocyst occur when the morula is floating in the uterine cavity. Eventually the zona pellucida disappears and the blastocyst becomes attached to the decidua, at the part of it overlying the inner cell mass (Figs 11, 13) and then sinks into the substance of the decidua. McLaren (1970) has shown that there are two factors contributing to the loss of the zona in mice; a lytic factor, which dissolves the zona and probably emanates from the uterus and the expansive activity of the blastocyst itself. When that occurs *implantation* commences and the earliest known normally implanted human

---

Fig. 12. Four early human embryos. The surface of the endometrium is to the right of the figure in each case.

A. An implanted early 9-day human blastocyst, seen towards the right of the figure. Syncytiotrophoblastic lacunae have formed, and one such lacuna is clearly shown in the upper part of the trophoblast. An amnion has developed, and the germ disc is still bilaminar. The endometrium is clearly secretory in character but a decidual reaction has not yet occurred. Carnegie 8215, 12-5-1. (× 75).

B. A 9-day implanted human blastocyst with features similar to those shown in A. The endometrium shows an early predecidual reaction with infiltrating leucocytes about the ovum. An empty maternal blood space in the upper part of the implantation site is communicating with coalescing lacunae of the blood space in the future intervillous space. Carnegie 8171, section 3-2-11. (× 75).

C. A mid cross-section of a 12-day human ovum showing an exocoelomic membrane and cavity of maximum size. The germ disc is bilaminar and the amnion and amniotic cavity well defined. The lacunar spaces intercommunicate and are filled with maternal blood. Early decidua is developing in the area immediately surrounding the ovum. Three irregular masses of cyto-trophoblast forming primordial villi project into the syncytium (at approximately 6 o'clock, 7 o'clock and 11 o'clock in the figure). The tall columnar ectodermal cells, and smaller endodermal cells of the embryonic disc are clearly visible. Carnegie 7700, section 6-1-5. (× 75).

D. A mid cross-section of a 12-day human ovum, demonstrating features similar to those shown in C. A primordial villus is present at about 6 o'clock in the figure. Carnegie 8330, section 9-2-6. (× 75).

blastocyst (Hertig and Rock, 1945) is 7½ days old (Figs 11, 12). Abnormally implantation can occur in the uterine tube or other sites, when an *ectopic gestation* results.

This process of implantation is very different in certain other mammals (Amoroso, 1952), particularly the ungulates, whose anatomy or physiological processes are often unique. In many ungulates the blastocyst may remain in the uterine cavity for several weeks before implantation and the uterine glands produce a copious secretion (uterine milk) in order to nourish the blastocyst in its sojourn inside the uterine cavity until it expands sufficiently

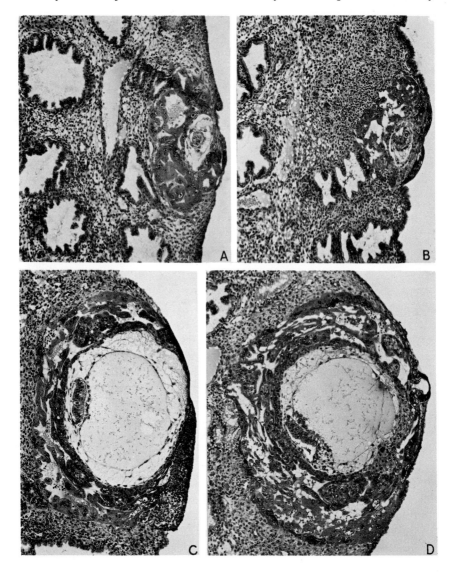

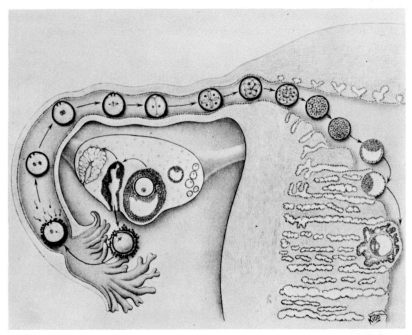

Fig. 13. Diagrammatic representation of the maturation of a Graafian follicle, ovulation and conversion of the collapsed follicle into a corpus luteum in the ovary. Fertilisation is seen occurring in the lateral portion of the uterine tube. As the fertilised ovum passes down the tube, it undergoes cleavage, forms a morula and then a blastocyst, which implants in the decidua.

to fill the uterine cavity so that the trophoblast becomes attached to the decidua.

The human blastocyst implants interstitially, i.e. below the surface of the decidua. The purpose of the secretory change in the uterine glands is to produce nourishment for the blastocyst before it implants, a type of nourishment called *histopoietic*. In effect the secretory change which occurs in the endometrium after ovulation is preparatory for the reception of a fertilized ovum. The trophoblast will not be concerned with the formation of any structure in the embryo itself; it forms only fetal membranes, including the placenta, and by its activity enables implantation to occur. The inner cell mass, on the other hand, is concerned solely with the production of embryonic tissue.

Development of germ layers

The first change to occur in the inner cell mass is that certain cells towards the segmentation cavity become segregated and cubical in shape, forming the *endoderm* of the embryo. These endoderm cells proliferate at the periphery of the inner cell mass and come to line the inside of the trophoblast to form a sac which is called the *primary yolk sac, exocoelomic membrane* or Heuser's membrane, which is homologous with the yolk sac of the reptiles. This homology has been taken as evidence of the reptilian origin of the mammals. The primary yolk sac is so called because it is later replaced by a true or definitive yolk sac. What actually happens is that endoderm cells continue to be proliferated from the periphery of the inner cell mass so that the primary yolk sac becomes too big for the blastocoele and buckles; eventually it is narrowed as the yolk sac duct which is then constricted off from the true or *secondary yolk sac* so that it lies in the segmentation cavity as an independent structure, atrophies and disappears (see Lewis and Harrison, 1966). This process is aided by the formation of extraembryonic mesoderm produced from the inner surface of the trophoblast. The secondary yolk sac is a very much smaller structure than the primary yolk sac and, while it is being formed, other changes are occurring in the inner cell mass and in the segmentation cavity which becomes filled with a loose reticulum of *extra-embryonic mesoderm,* called *magma reticulare,* formed from the inner surface of the trophoblast. As already mentioned, the proliferation of these extraembryonic mesoderm cells pushes the primary yolk sac away from the trophoblast (it is possible that the primary yolk sac also develops from the inner surface of the cytotrophoblast (see Fig. 12 and Hertig, Rock and Adams, 1956) rather than from the endoderm of the embryonic disc), so that eventually it shrivels and atrophies, thus restricting the secondary yolk sac to a small area in the region of the inner cell mass. A cavity soon appears amongst the cells of the inner cell mass, which is called the *amniotic cavity.* It is covered over by cells forming the amniotic membrane or *amnion,* derived partly from the inner cell mass and partly from "amniogenic" cells of the trophoblast immediately overlying the inner cell mass; the cells in the floor of the amniotic cavity become tall and columnar and form the *ectoderm.* This process results in the establishment of an embryonic disc which is composed of columnar ectodermal cells in the floor of the amniotic cavity lying above the cubical endodermal cells which are themselves in the roof of the yolk sac. While this change is occurring, the extraembryonic mesoderm fills up the whole of the segmentation cavity, but soon a cavity appears in it called the extraembryonic coelom, which separates the cells of the extraembryonic mesoderm into two layers; one layer lines the inside of the trophoblast and is called *somatopleuric extraembryonic mesoderm,* while the other is applied to the outside of the yolk sac and is called *splanchnopleuric extraembryonic mesoderm.* The extraembryonic mesoderm in contact with the amnion is also called somatopleuric. The somatopleuric extraembryonic mesoderm plus the trophoblast constitute a membrane called the *chorion.* The amnion and the chorion are fetal membranes, which together cover the developing fetus right up to the time of parturition. In fact the membranes normally rupture to allow the baby to be born. If not, then the baby is born in its membranes and this is colloquially termed "being born in a caul". The amniotic sac contains amniotic fluid, whose volume increases throughout pregnancy (Harrison and Malpas, 1953); it provides a fluid environment for all developing *amniotes* (animals possessing an amniotic sac) which enabled emancipation from aquatic surroundings, during the evolutionary process. As the amnion grows the somatopleuric extraembryonic mesoderm covering it is increasingly brought into contact with the chorion, thus obliterating most of the extraembryonic coelom. A chorio-amniotic membrane is thus created, through which material from maternal vessels in the decidua parietalis can diffuse into the amniotic fluid and vice versa.

Hertig, Rock and Adams (1956) have described 34 human ova within the first 17 days of development and provide an excellent record of the changes during this period. They have also shown that abnormalities develop and are recognisable in embryos at such an early stage of development; this has been confirmed by Harrison, Hilton Jones and Parry Jones (1966) who found abnormal features, such as malorientation of the embryonic disc and excessive mitotic activity, in a human embryo aged 13 days.

CLINICAL RELATIONSHIPS

The danger of an ectopic gestation occurring in the uterine tube is related to the inability of the relatively thin wall of the tube to sustain a growing conceptus. Frequently the pregnancy terminates at the second or third month by rupture of the tube, a severe haemorrhage into the peritoneal cavity and death of the embryo. The shock resulting from the blood loss may be sufficiently severe as to endanger the life of the mother, and such a ruptured tubal pregnancy constitutes an obstetric emergency. On the other hand, erosion of the tubal wall may be more "silent", the chorionic vesicle passing through it without noticeable symptoms, and establishing secondary implantation on the peritoneum, usually peritoneum surrounding the alimentary canal.

The child resulting from such a pregnancy obviously cannot be born *per vias naturales,* and must be delivered by abdominal operation. Pregnancy can occur in the ovary; when it occurs as a result of fertilization of the oocyte before it leaves the ovary this is a primary ovarian pregnancy. Some clinicians maintain, however, that all ovarian pregnancies are secondary to a ruptured tubal pregnancy. A tubal pregnancy usually occurs because of obstruction to the passage of the fertilized ovum along the uterine tube by adhesions resulting from previous infection (e.g. gonorrhoea) and chronic inflammation of the tube (see Harrison and de Boer, 1976). An interstitial pregnancy occurs when implantation takes place in the intramural part of the uterine tube—the terminal portion where it traverses the uterine wall; it usually terminates in abortion.

In the macaque monkey, implantation occurs at more than one site. After the primary implantation, as the chorionic vesicle enlarges and contacts other parts of the uterine decidua, other sites of attachment and the development of implantation sites occurs. Similar attachment in more than one site may occur in human implantation so that it is possible for the placenta to have two or more lobes of more or less equal size (placenta duplex, triplex or multiplex) each with its own umbilical vessels. In like fashion there may develop a main placenta with one or two separate small accessory lobes, supplied by branches of umbilical vessels from the main placenta. This is known as succenturiate placenta. If the separation of the lobes is incomplete, bipartite or tripartite placenta results. All of these conditions of the placenta are of importance, since it is clearly possible for one or other of the smaller lobes to be left in the uterus during the third stage of labour, with resultant post-partum haemorrhage.

Amniotic fluid variations

The volume of amniotic fluid increases throughout pregnancy until about the 32nd week, when it begins to fall as parturition approaches. This fall has been interpreted as a factor in the initiation of parturition, since disturbance of the normal relationships that exist between intrauterine pressure, tension per unit area of uterine wall and the radius of the uterus, are known to facilitate myometrial contractions. The source of origin of the amniotic fluid varies throughout pregnancy. Thus, in the early stages the amnion itself may be concerned, fluid being secreted from the amnion, particularly that on the fetal surface of the placenta. When the kidneys of the fetus begin to function they excrete urine into the amniotic fluid, and it is also known that fetuses are able to swallow their own amniotic fluid. In late fetal life, respiratory-like movements cause amniotic fluid to be drawn into the fetal lungs, and this is undoubtedly a factor assisting their development. The volume of amniotic fluid at full term is approximately 500-800 ml.

An increase in the amount of amniotic fluid beyond 2 litres is definitely abnormal, and described as hydramnios. Such a condition occurs in certain abnormalities of the fetus. Thus, when the fetus is unable to swallow, as for example when the oesophagus shows atresia, or if, as in the anencephalic child, there is lack of the normal nervous control of swallowing, hydramnios regularly occurs. It has also been suggested that the exposed choroid plexuses in anencephaly may be a factor in increasing the volume of amniotic fluid by secretion from the plexuses. On the other hand, in agenesis of the kidneys, or if a fetus develops atresia of the urethra, the amount of amniotic fluid is decreased (oligoamnios).

The fact that it is possible to remove 10-15 ml amniotic fluid by amniocentesis, a procedure in which a needle is inserted through the abdominal wall into the amniotic cavity, avoiding the placenta, has made possible the prenatal diagnosis of fetal anomalies. Thus, the presence of elevated a-fetoprotein levels in the amniotic fluid points to the leakage of fetal blood into the fluid from open defects in the body surface in cases of anencephaly or spina bifida (see p. 63). Since the fluid also contains many cells exfoliated from the amnion and the fetus, these can be grown in tissue culture and then examined for any chromosome abnormalities. Thus Down's Syndrome can be detected before birth and a selective abortion performed.

References

Amoroso, E. C. (1952). *In* "Marshall's Physiology of Reproduction" Vol. II. 3rd Edn. Chap. 15, pp. 127-311. Longmans Green, London.

Austin, C. R. and Bishop, M. W. H. (1957). Fertilization in mammals. *Biol. Rev.* **32,** 296.

Corner, G. W. (1944). "Ourselves Unborn" Yale Univ. Press, New Haven.

Harrison, R. G. and de Boer (1976). "Sex and Infertility" Academic Press, London.

Harrison, R. G. and Malpas, P. (1953). The volume of human amniotic fluid. *J. Obstet. Gynaec. Br. Gommonw.* **60,** 631-638.

Harrison, R. G., Jones, C. Hilton and Jones, E. Parry (1966). A pathological presomite human embryo. *J. Path. Bact.* **92,** 583-584.

Hertig, A. T. and Rock, J. (1945). Two human ova of the pre-villous stage, having a developmental age of about seven and nine days respectively. *Contr. Embryol.* **31,** 65-84.

Hertig, A. T. and Rock, J. (1951). The implantation and early development of the human ovum. *Am. J. Obstet. Gynec.* **61,** 8-14.

Hertig, A. T., Rock, J. and Adams, E. C. (1956). A description of 34 human ova within the first 17 days of development. *Am. J. Anat.* **98,** 435-494.

Hertig, A. T., Rock, J., Adams, E. C. and Mulligan, W. J. (1954). On the preimplantation stages of the human ovum: a description of four normal and four abnormal specimens ranging from the second to the fifth day of development. *Contr. Embryol.* **35,** 199-220.

Heuser, C. H. and Streeter, G. L. (1941). Development of the macaque embryo. *Contr. Embryol.* **29,** 15-55.

Lewis, B. V. and Harrison, R. G. (1966). A presomite human embryo showing a yolk-sac duct. *J. Anat.* **100,** 389-396.

McLaren, A. (1970). The fate of the zona pellucida in mice. *J. Embryol. Exp. Morphol.* **23,** 1-19.

Rothschild, Lord (1956). "Fertilization" Methuen, London.

5

The Development of the Placenta

Before implantation the zona pellucida must disappear in order that the trophoblast cells of the blastocyst can become stuck on to the inner surface of the decidua; the attachment always occurs in the region overlying the inner cell mass. The earliest known implanted human blastocyst is 7½ days old and the attachment to the decidua before actual implantation probably occurs some time between 4½ and 7 days (Hertig, Rock and Adams, 1956). During the next two or three days the blastocyst sinks into the decidua, which eventually covers over its surface; the manner of this interstitial implantation is quite characteristic of the human being and involves the cells of the surface of the blastocyst, namely the trophoblast, which proliferate most actively at this time. Enzymes are produced by the cells of the trophoblast, which begin to erode the decidua and this aids the interstitial implantation of the blastocyst. In other words, there is a digestion of the maternal tissue by the trophoblast and the pabulum of digested decidua passes across the tropho-blast wall into the blastocoele, and serves to nourish the growing embryo by *histolytic* nutrition. The implantation occurs rapidly (in fact by the 10th day the blastocyst is completely implanted below the surface of the decidua) and the proliferation of the trophoblast forms two types of cell. The first is called the *cytotrophoblast* since its constituent cells are clearly demarcated from one another. The cytotrophoblastic cells divide to form a further layer of cells on their surface which fuse together to form a syncytium. This outer syncytial layer of trophoblast is therefore termed the *syncytiotrophoblast;* evidence of the fact that it is formed by fusion of its constituent cells is shown by the persistence of parts of the cell boundaries in between the cells clearly visible on electron microscopy (see Boyd and Hamilton, 1970).

The Liverpool embryo, 16 days old (Harrison and Jeffcoate, 1953), shows these layers of cells very clearly and the site through which the blastocyst breaches the epithelium to become implanted inside the decidua, which becomes closed over by a plug of fibrin, called the fibrin plug or closing plug (Fig. 14). As the trophoblast proliferates, finger-like processes (villi) are pushed out from the surface of the blastocyst; these trophoblastic villi are first of all composed only of syncytiotrophoblast and cytotrophoblast. Later, somatopleuric extraembryonic mesoderm grows into the villi. A villus which consists only of cytotrophoblast and syncytiotrophoblast is called a primary villus. One also containing somatopleuric extraembryonic mesoderm is called a secondary villus; a tertiary villus is formed at a much later stage, when the embryo is completely implanted and blood vessels, which grow into the connecting stalk (which will form the umbilical cord), run into the extraembryonic mesoderm of the villi. When extraembryonic mesoderm grows into the villi, they are termed *chorionic villi.* The uterine decidua can be divided into three main types according to its situation. That which is lying in contact with the blastocyst at the site of implantation is called the *decidua basalis;* the decidua which covers over the surface of the implanting blastocyst is called the *decidua capsularis,* while the remainder of the decidua lining the inside of the uterus is called the *decidua parietalis* or decidua vera (Fig. 15). The decidua basalis helps to form the placenta, the localized discoidal structure, formed at the site of implantation from the decidua basalis and the chorionic villi.

Chorionic development

Although originally the trophoblastic villi develop all over the surface of the blastocyst, at one stage they cease to be produced and degenerate completely

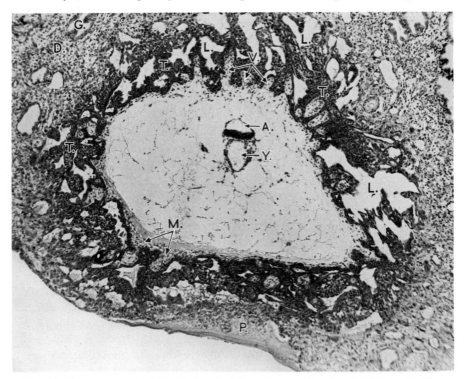

Fig. 14. Photomicrograph of the blastocyst of the "Liverpool I embryo", 16 days old. The blastocyst has implanted into the decidua, and the site of implantation is closed by the fibrin plug (P.). The trophoblast (T.) is forming villi (V.), containing extraembryonic mesoderm (M.), which are pushing into the decidual stroma (D.). Lacunae (L.) have formed in the trophoblast, and at least one of the decidual glands (G.) is visible. The amniotic cavity (A.), and yolk sac (Y.), between which is the bilaminar embryonic disc, are visible. The blastocoele is filled with magma reticulare. ($\times$ 56).

everywhere except at the embryonic pole of the blastocyst, so leaving the surface of the chorion in contact with the decidua capsularis quite smooth (the *chorion laeve*), whereas the villi towards the decidua basalis grow, proliferate and become much more complicated (the *chorion frondosum*). Only the chorion frondosum participates in the formation of the true placenta; the mature placenta, therefore, consists of two parts, the uterine

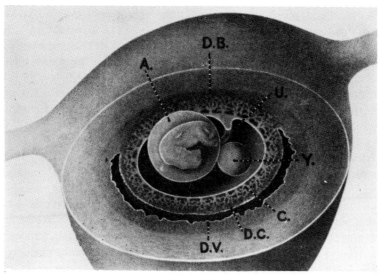

Fig. 15. Diagrammatic representation of the pregnant uterus showing the decidua basalis (D.B.), decidua capsularis (D.C.), and decidua vera (D.V.). The embryo is inside the amniotic cavity (A.) and attached to the chorion (C.), whose villi are clearly shown, by the body stalk (U.). The yolk sac (Y.) is also visible.

part of the placenta which is formed from the decidua basalis and the fetal placenta developed from the chorion frondosum. As the syncytiotrophoblast grows, cavities formed by coalescence of smaller vacuoles, called *lacunae* (see Wislocki and Bennett, 1943), appear. These vacuoles are probably an expression of metabolic exchange. The lacunae are therefore separated from one another by syncytiotrophoblastic trabeculae. As early as the twelfth day the majority of lacunae have come into free communication with one another and the earliest villi, in fact, consist of the trabeculae which persist in between the lacunae. The confluence of the lacunae in the early placenta, therefore, brings into being the *intervillous space*. As the syncytiotrophoblast proliferates and grows into the decidua, it breaches the uterine vessels. The walls of the uterine blood vessels break down and, therefore, blood escapes from them into the intervillous space. The primary villi formed from the trabeculae therefore pass from the chorion on the fetal side of the intervillous space—*the chorionic plate*—to the maternal decidua basalis. From each primary villus is formed the *truncus chorii,* or main stem villus, from which smaller *rami chorii* branch and these in turn branch to form the *ramuli chorii* from which chorionic villi are suspended in the maternal blood of the intervillous space, and when the fetal blood vessels grow into the chorionic villi it is therefore possible for amino acids, fatty acids, glucose, mineral salts and water to be supplied from the maternal to the fetal circulations. Waste material and carbon dioxide pass in the reverse direction.

There is never, however, any continuity between the uterine and fetal circulations; a membrane formed by the walls of the chorionic villi always separates them. The trunci chorii which pass from the chorionic plate of the placenta across the intervillous space to be attached to the decidua basalis act as anchoring villi. The majority of villi, however, hang floating freely in the intervillous space not attached to the decidua basalis. From the points where the trunci chorii reach and anchor onto the decidua basalis, cyto-trophoblast spreads out over its inner surface as the cytotrophoblastic shell. Backward projections of trophoblast from this shell grow into the intervillous space to form *septa,* which divide the fetal part of the placenta into 10 to 38 areas called *lobes* or *cotyledons,* each containing several trunci chorii and the villi which branch out from them (Fig. 16). These cotyledons are very obvious on the uterine surface of the mature placenta. The cytotrophoblastic shell, together with the decidua basalis on which it lies, constitutes the *basal plate* of the placenta. The basal plate is therefore the site of junction between the maternal and fetal tissues and is perforated by the maternal blood vessels passing to and from the intervillous space.

Immunological relationships

The extensive degree of fusion of chorionic tissue containing the fetal blood vessels with the decidua basalis is of great interest, since fetal tissue can set up an *antigen-antibody* response in the maternal organism. One of the best known examples of such a phenomenon is the incompatibility of Rh blood groups in fetus and mother when a Rhesus positive fetus causes the production of antibodies in a Rhesus negative mother: these antibodies then pass across the placenta from maternal to fetal circulations and produce a haemolytic disease in the fetus. It is known that the permeability of the placenta to different substances probably varies according to their molecular size. Thus the virus of rubella can cross the placenta into the foetal circulation but more recently it has been found that both maternal and fetal blood corpuscles can traverse the placenta into the opposite circulation. This phenomenon would, at first sight, appear to require some damage to the tissue layers separating the maternal and fetal circulations. It is known that the number of such layers diminishes towards the end of pregnancy; the cytotrophoblastic cells in the villi diminish or even disappear entirely and the syncytiotrophoblast becomes much thinner. Coincidentally there is, from as early as the third month of fetal life, a deposition of fibrin and fibrinoid material in both the basal plate ("Nitabuch's stria") and chorionic plate and in the septa. All these changes have been interpreted as an ageing process in the placenta but they must clearly lead to alterations in the permeability of

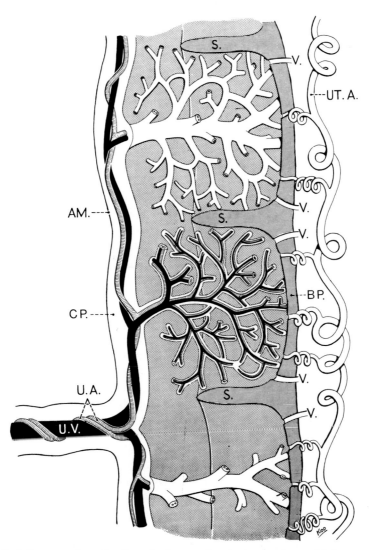

Fig. 16. A diagrammatic section through a human placenta showing three cotyledons separated by septa (S.). In each cotyledon is shown a truncus chorii, passing from the chorionic plate (CP.) across the intervillous space to be anchored to the basal plate (BP.). The truncus has rami and ramuli chorii branching off from it. The uterine artery (UT.A.) is seen giving off spiral branches into the intervillous space which is drained by veins (V.) at its periphery. The umbilical cord with umbilical arteries (U.A.) and umbilical vein (U.V.) is seen approaching the fetal surface of the placenta which is covered by amnion (AM.). (Modified from Hamilton and Boyd, 1960).

the placenta. Whether there is normally any actual damage or disappearance of tissue in the villi to an extent allowing dissolution of fetal tissue and resultant communication between the two circulations, is still not clearly established. Nevertheless, it has been shown that the cells of the syncytio-trophoblast have microvilli, a large number of organelles, pinosomes, vesicles and canaliculi, in addition to other cellular inclusions and substances such as lipids and carbohydrates. Pinocytosis by syncytiotrophoblastic cells is known to occur from early in pregnancy and it is therefore conceivable that substances of large molecular size, even blood corpuscles, may be passed across the placental barrier as a result of phagocytosis, or some similar mechanism, by these cells.

Because of fusion between the maternal decidua basalis and the fetal cytotrophoblastic shell, the basal plate of the placenta is a region where immunological phenomena are located, in addition to the overall immuno-logical manifestations occurring between mother and fetus and witnessed particularly in such cases as Rh incompatibility. The placenta itself, together with the fetus, may be considered as a special type of graft, with genetic endowment from both mother and father; they constitute an isograft in relation to the mother and a homograft in respect of the father. Some immunological reaction might be expected, therefore, and this may damage the embryo or placenta, perhaps even resulting in their expulsion from the uterus. Many investigators have attempted to determine why such rejection of the embryo and placenta does not occur and one of the factors concerned may be the increasing deposition of fibrin and fibrinoid in the basal plate as pregnancy advances. However, the barrier constituted by this fibrin is not complete and other features must be implicated, the most likely being the absence of antigenicity in the trophoblast. It has also been suggested that the uterus is an "Immunologically privileged site", a site in which an allograft fails to elicit, or is protected against, an immune response and that this is brought about by an absence of lymphatics in the endometrium (McLean and Scothorne, 1970).

Although transmission of immunity in monkeys and Man appears to be mainly by way of the chorioallantoic placenta (p. 51), it is possible that some maternal antibody reaches the fetus by way of the amniotic cavity and fetal gut (Brambell, 1970). It should be remembered that transmission also occurs after birth by secretion in the colostrum (the fluid secreted by the mammary gland a few days before and after parturition) and milk and subsequent absorption by the neonatal gut. The colostrum of those species in which transmission occurs after birth is characterized by its high content of immunoglobulins, in contrast to those species in which such transmission does not occur.

There is a remarkable selective transmission of immunity in many species: certainly before birth in Man. Selection in all cases operates in favour of homologous γ-globulin as compared to the other proteins of homologous serum, and in most cases in favour of γ-globulin as compared to the other proteins of a heterologous serum. There is also clear evidence of selection between the various components of γ-globulin; for example, γ M-globulin is transmitted from mother to fetus in the rabbit but not in Man. In most species and probably in all, serum albumin is transmitted at the same time as the γ-globulin, though less readily. On the other hand, the available evidence suggests that the passage of maternal proteins to the human amniotic fluid may be non-selective.

The mature placenta

The type of placenta varies in the different mammalian orders and even between species; that in the human is called haemochorial because maternal blood is in direct contact with the chorion. It is termed villous because it has chorionic villi and it is also deciduate, because there is shedding of decidua at parturition. The fetal surface of the placenta is connected to the embryo by a band of somatopleuric extraembryonic mesoderm, the body stalk, and when blood vessels pass from the embryo to the placenta they grow in the body stalk and so convert it into the umbilical cord, so called because it attaches the placenta to the fetal umbilicus. This cord normally contains two umbilical arteries but only one umbilical vein during the greater part of pregnancy. In the early embryo, there are two umbilical veins but later one of these (the right) atrophies. The branches of the uterine arteries (which are spiral) empty into the intervillous spaces at the centre of each cotyledon (Bøe, 1952). Hamilton and Boyd (1960) have shown that the spiral arteries do not open directly into the intervillous space; the maternal blood first percolates through intercellular gaps in the trophoblastic shell and leaves it through randomly distributed venous openings. Ramsey (1954) has reviewed the venous drainage of the placenta; she shows that the classic arrangement proposed by Spanner is probably inaccurate and that the views of Stieve are more likely. Spanner lays great stress on the *marginal sinus,* a prolongation of the lake of blood lying in the intervillous space into the edge (margin) of the placenta where placenta tapers off and the chorion and amnion become applied to the decidua vera; he asserted that the venous drainage of the mature placenta is effected exclusively through the marginal sinus and that other veins draining the intervillous space in young placentae are later obliterated. Stieve claimed that branches of the uterine veins open all over the uterine surface of the placenta and averred that the marginal sinus is not present in the normal placenta, a view which has been confirmed (Hamilton and Boyd, 1951).

The mature placenta is 10 to 24 cm in diameter, about 3 cm thick at its centre and weighs about 500 g. The usual arrangement is for the umbilical cord to be attached to the centre (i.e. central attachment of the umbilical cord). It may, however, be attached at the periphery of the placenta—a condition called battledore placenta—or even to the fetal membranes at a point slightly removed from the edge of the placenta, a condition called velamentous insertion of the cord. It is also possible for there to be an accessory lobe of the placenta—the succenturiate lobe. Because the placenta is formed from that part of the chorion which continued to develop as the chorion frondosum, it can be seen how the remainder of the chorion is continuous with the margins of the placenta. The placenta normally develops on the anterior or posterior wall of the uterus but it can develop near the cervix, sometimes even overlapping it, a condition called *placenta praevia*. As the blastocyst enlarges, it fills the whole of the uterine cavity so pushing in front of it the decidua capsularis, which contacts and fuses with the decidua vera. The amnion also enlarges, so that eventually the amniotic cavity fills the inside of the segmentation cavity and obliterates it. The embryo comes to lie inside the amniotic cavity and is suspended in the fluid environment of it by the umbilical cord. The tissues surrounding the fetus are therefore now established; from without inwards they are the decidua, then the chorion and finally the amnion. The chorion and amnion are *fetal membranes*.

CLINICAL RELATIONSHIPS

At any given age, there is great variability in human placental weight and, indeed, in that of the associated embryo or fetus (Boyd and Hamilton, 1970). This is due to three factors. First, there may be variations in the amount of tissue, fetal and decidual, which separate during dehiscence of the placenta. Second, there may be variations in the amount of blood or blood clot in the placenta. Thirdly, different observers may include varying amounts of membranes or umbilical cord in their measurements. It is, however, very clear that the rate of placental growth is not as rapid as that of the fetus. An increase in fetal weight of 100 g is accompanied by an increase in placental weight of 12·7 g. This discrepancy in growth rates may be due to the fact that some exchange of materials between fetus and mother can take place other than through the chorio-allantoic placenta (e.g. across the chorio-amniotic membrane, see pp. 34, 51). At term the weight of the placenta is about 14% that of fetal weight.

The placenta is an organ of gas as well as nutritional exchange, and itself has a far from negligible oxygen consumption (see Dawes, 1968). For the physiologist and the obstetrician, it is important to know the directions and velocities of blood flow on both sides of the placental membrane separating maternal and fetal blood, the quantitative features of the membrane (e.g. its surface area) and the structure of the membrane and any variations which may occur in it with gestational age and disease. As pregnancy advances, the syncytiotrophoblast becomes thinner and the cytotrophoblast largely disappears, persisting only as isolated cells in the terminal villi. The trophoblastic basement membrane may, however, thicken in the last few weeks of pregnancy, and deposits of fibrin and a related substance termed fibrinoid accumulate in placental structures. Thus in the normal placenta fibrin appears in the chorionic plate (Langhan's fibrin stria) and fibrinoid is found in the basal plate (the striae of Rohr and Nitabuch). Fibrinoid is a precipitate of acid mucopolysaccharides in the ground substance of the tissues concerned. The accumulation of fibrin and fibrinoid within the placenta has been taken as evidence of "ageing" of the placenta by some investigators; but such normal accumulations should be distinguished from "white infarcts" which are produced by ischaemia of parts of the placenta, resulting from coagulation of blood around chorionic villi. The infarct is at first red, owing to engorgement of blood within the villi, but later becomes fibrosed and white. The greater the infarct, the more extensive the interference with placental function and the danger to fetal life; a massive infarct may be found in more than 50% of placentas at full term.

There is, however, normally an enhancement of the functional efficiency of the human placenta (in terms of diffusion of materials across it) as pregnancy advances, not only as a result of thinning of the placental membrane, but also because of a decrease in diameter of individual villi and an increase in the total number of terminal villi in the course of placental maturation; the capillaries within each villus increase in number and become more closely applied to the surface of the villus wall.

The umbilical cord

The umbilical cord is very variable in length, from 2·3 cm at three months to 48 cm at term (Boyd and Hamilton, 1970). Malpas (1964) has recorded variations in length of the full-term cord from 30 to 129 cm (mean length 61 cm); he suggested that such variability is compatible with normal fetal growth, and may be explained by the umbilical blood vessels growing in one dimension only. Nevertheless, an abnormally long cord may twist around the neck of the fetus, as a result of fetal movement in utero, and during parturition or even before birth, if the cord is tightly wound, the babe may strangle itself with its own cord. The umbilical blood vessels in the cord are usually twisted around one another, the helices being sinistral rather than dextral and varying in number from 0 to 380. The twists must be distinguished from periodic partial constrictions ("Valves of Hoboken") in the umbilical arteries. These are not really valves and have been variously interpreted as folds or cushions resulting from contraction of the tunica media of the arteries, or simply thinning of the arterial wall in between the "valves". "True" and "false" knots can occur in the cord. True knots, like twisting of the cord round the neck, can cause intrauterine death of the fetus. False knots are associated with atypical looping of umbilical vessels, a localized dilation of the umbilical vein, or a nodal accumulation of Wharton's jelly, the specialized connective tissue formed from extraembryonic mesoderm which surrounds the vessels. One umbilical artery may be absent in 1% cases and is closely associated with a high incidence of congenital fetal anomalies.

Just before entering the chorionic plate the two umbilical arteries are joined by fusion with one another, by a secondary opening or most commonly (90% cases) by a transverse branch between them (Hyrtl's anastomosis). The two arteries then separate and branch in a variety of patterns—mostly dichotomously (the "disperse" type). It has been suggested that if the arteries extend almost to the margin of the placenta before division (the "magistral" type) this favours better fetal development by providing more ideal haemodynamic conditions for blood supply of the placenta.

Hormonal secretion by placenta

One important feature about the placenta is that it secretes oestrogenic hormones, progesterone, and a hormone peculiar to the placenta, chorionic gonadotrophin. These hormones are probably produced by the syncytio-trophoblast, as shown by histochemical observations and the localization of several enzymes whose action is primarily steroidogenic. When the placenta becomes fully established it produces progesterone in sufficient amounts to maintain the pregnancy, and when this occurs at about the third month of pregnancy, it is no longer necessary for the corpora lutea to secrete this hormone and they degenerate; as a result both of the ovaries can be removed with impunity after the third month (see Courrier, 1945). Before the third month, however, bilateral ovariectomy would produce an abortion. Although the cortex of the suprarenal glands secretes progesterone, the amount is small and probably plays an insignificant role in the maintenance of pregnancy.

Oestrogenic hormones are secreted in increasing amounts during pregnancy, reaching a maximum just before birth, and indeed the rise at this time may, in part, be responsible for the onset of parturition (see Reynolds, 1949). Chorionic gonadotrophin is secreted as soon as the chorion itself is formed, and therefore the excretion of this hormone in the urine can be utilized as a test for pregnancy. Chorionic gonadotrophin has a luteinizing action; in other words, it is very similar in its effect to that of L.H. of the anterior lobe of the pituitary gland. Therefore if chorionic gonadotrophin or the urine from a pregnant woman is injected into an immature mouse, corporea lutea will be formed, and this is the basis of the Aschheim-Zondek test for pregnancy. A similar test can be performed on a rabbit, the Friedman test, but even more rapid than either of these is the pregnancy test using the South African toad Xenopus laevis. If this is treated with the urine from a pregnant woman, the toad ovulates. Still more rapid than this, however, is the Galli-Mainini test which employs the male frog; if urine from a pregnant woman is injected into its dorsal lymph sac spermatozoa appear in the frog's urine within 48 hours. Since 1960 these biological tests have been supplanted by *in vitro* immunological techniques which depend on the observation that, in the presence of human pregnancy urine, sheep red-cells or latex particles sensitized with human chorionic gonadotrophin (H.C.G.) are not agglutinated by antiserum to H.C.G.

Comparative placentation. Placenta as allograft

It should be stressed that the manner of implantation in the human is highly specialized. The authoritative works of Amoroso (1952) and Steven (1975) should be consulted for the mechanism of implantation and placentation in other mammals. Borland (1975) has recently summarized the function of the placenta as an allograft (a graft of tissue between different individuals of the same species). The fetus, fetal membranes and placenta together constitute a peculiarly successful allograft, for the conceptus not only survives but also develops in a hostile environment. The success is due to the development of a fetal-maternal barrier intimately associated with the trophoblast cell layer. This barrier is in large part composed of chorionic gonadotrophin which has sialic acid as part of its molecule, or it is formed as a result of "immunological enhancement" and may consist of serum a- and β-glycoproteins having sialic acids associated with the molecule, which interact with conventional antibodies to provide a protective coat around foreign cells, so that they can survive.

Hydatidiform mole. Chorion-epithelioma

Excessive, unregulated proliferation of trophoblast tissue results in a chorionic sac covered with a large number of fluid-filled vesicles, a condition termed hydatidiform mole. This condition, which is associated with fetal death, is to be considered as a benign tumour and must be removed from the uterus, since there is always the danger of malignancy supervening (chorion-epithelioma). As might be expected, the quantity of chorionic gonadotrophin secreted in such cases is greater than normal, excessive in chorion-epithelioma, and this allows for their detection.

Single artery cords

In about 1% of umbilical cords, one of the arteries is absent, and there is a great deal of evidence to suggest that this is associated with the presence of congenital malformations in the fetus (Armitage et al., 1967). All fetal organ systems are equally prone to the associated anomalies, though there is a slight preponderance for genito-urinary defects. There is a higher percentage of placental abnormalities in cases of absence of one cord artery. A single artery is commoner in monozygotic twins than in singleton pregnancy, and there seems to be an association between umbilical artery aplasia and trisomy excluding cases of Down's syndrome.

References

Amoroso, E. C. (1952). In "Marshall's Physiology of Reproduction" Vol. II. 3rd Edn. Chap. 15, p. 127. Longmans Green, London.

Armitage, P., Boyd, J. D., Hamilton, W. J. and Rowe, B. C. (1967). A statistical analysis of a series of birth-weights and placental weights. Hum. Biol. **39**, 430-444.

Bøe, S. (1952). Studies on the vascularization of the human placenta. Acta obstet. gynec. scand. **32**, Suppl. 5, 1-92.

Borland, R. (1975). *In* "Comparative Placentation" (Ed. D. H. Steven) Chap. 9, p. 268. Academic Press, London.

Boyd, J. D. and Hamilton, W. J. (1970). "The Human Placenta" Heffer, Cambridge.

Brambell, F. W. Rogers (1970). "The Transmission of Passive Immunity from Mother to Young" North Holland, London.

Courrier, R. (1945). "Endocrinologie de la Gestation" Masson, Paris.

Dawes, A. (1968). "Foetal and Neonatal Physiology" Year Book Medical Publisher's, Chicago.

Hamilton, W. J. and Boyd, J. D. (1951). Observations on the human placenta. *Proc. R. Soc. Med.* **44**, 489-496.

Hamilton, W. J. and Boyd, J. D. (1960). Development of the human placenta in the first three months of gestation. *J. Anat.* **94**, 297-328.

Harrison, R. G. and Jeffcoate, T. N. A. (1953). A presomite human embryo showing an early stage of the primitive streak. *J. Anat.* **87**, 124-129.

Hertig, A. T., Rock, J. and Adams, E. C. (1956). A description of 34 human ova within the first 17 days of development. *Am. J. Anat.* **98**, 435-494.

Malpas, P. (1964). Length of the human umbilical cord at term. *Brit. Med. J.* **1**, 673-674.

McLean, J. M. and Scothorne, R. J. (1970). The lymphatics of the endometrium in the rabbit. *J. Anat.* **107**, 39-48.

Ramsey, E. M. (1954). Circulation in the maternal placenta of primates. *Amer. J. Obstet. Gynec.* **67**, 1-14.

Reynolds, S. R. M. (1949). "Physiology of the Uterus" 2nd Edn. Hoeber, New York.

Steven, D. H. (1975). "Comparative Placentation" Academic Press, London.

Wislocki, G. B. and Bennett, H. S. (1943). Histology and cytology of the human and monkey placenta, with special reference to the trophoblast. *Am. J. Anat.* **73**, 335-449.

6

Flexion of the Embryo

Early differentiation

At the stage when the young embryo has an amniotic cavity and a true secondary yolk sac, the embryonic plate lying between the two cavities is bilaminar, consisting of ectoderm and endoderm only. Soon the ectodermal cells at the future caudal end of the embryonic plate assume pluripotential properties; they proliferate and form the *primitive streak* which is able to form not only new ectoderm and endoderm, but also *intraembryonic mesoderm,* which grows out at first laterally in between the ectoderm and endoderm, thus producing a trilaminar embryonic plate. At the cephalic end of the primitive streak a small proliferation of cells produces a node— Hensen's node—from which a cord of cells grows cephalically in the axis of the embryonic plate in between the ectoderm and endoderm. This is the *notochordal process*—it does not quite reach the extreme anterior end of the embryonic plate in its growth cephalically, for it is stopped at the caudal end of a region called the *prochordal plate* where ectoderm and endoderm are in such intimate contact that the notochordal process cannot separate them (Fig. 17). Immediately in front of the prochordal plate is an area of intraembryonic mesoderm called the *protocardiac area.* The intraembryonic mesoderm which is produced from the primitive streak at the caudal end of the embryonic plate migrates out not only laterally but also cephalically in between the ectoderm and endoderm—it comes to lie everywhere in the embryonic plate lateral to the notochordal process (which by now has differentiated into the true notochord, after canalization and intercalation with the endoderm) but is found in the mid-line only in the protocardiac area. Since it passes out laterally to the edge of the embryonic plate it will there meet the extraembryonic mesoderm, as can be seen in a transverse section of the embryo at this stage (Fig. 18). Immediately overlying the notochord there is a thickening of the ectoderm which is called the *medullary* or *neural plate,* the lateral margins of which rise up to form folds, the *neural folds,* in between which is the *neural groove*—these eventually meet and fuse to form a tube, the *neural tube,* over the top of which the ectoderm re-establishes continuity.

A longitudinal section through the embryo at this stage (Fig. 17) shows the neural plate and in front of this the protocardiac mesoderm; immediately in front of this is a collection of intraembryonic mesoderm called the *septum transversum.* Behind the neural plate is the blastopore, which lies in Hensen's node and indicates the site from which the notochordal process is

49

canalized prior to its intercalation with the endoderm and eventual solidification to form the true notochord. Behind the blastopore is the primitive streak, and because this is an actively dividing area producing intra-embryonic mesoderm it bulges into the amniotic cavity.

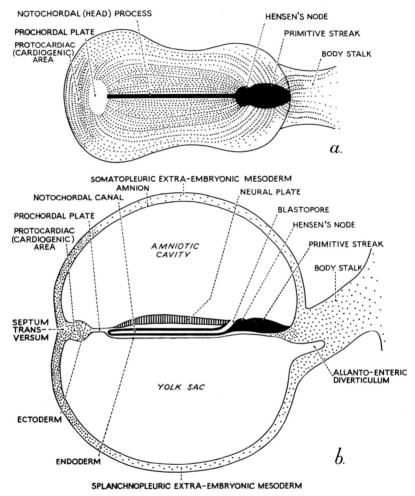

Fig. 17. Diagrammatic representation of the human embryo at the stage of the bilaminar embryonic plate seen from the dorsal aspect (a.) and in longitudinal section (b.). Mesoderm is shown in stipple.

Allanto-enteric diverticulum

The caudal end of the yolk sac forms a small diverticulum called the allanto-enteric diverticulum; this pushes into the region of the body stalk, which itself is continuous with the somatopleuric extraembryonic mesoderm overlying the amniotic cavity on the one hand, and the splanchnopleuric extraembryonic mesoderm covering the yolk sac on the other, both of which at the cephalic end of the embryo are continuous with the intraembryonic mesoderm of the septum transversum and protocardiac mesoderm and, at the lateral margins of the embryonic plate, with the intraembryonic mesoderm lying in between the ectoderm and endoderm. The allanto-enteric diver-

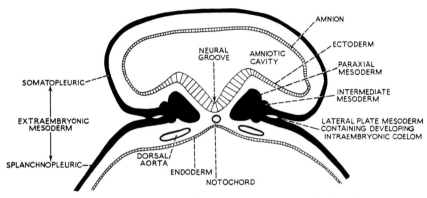

Fig. 18. Diagrammatic transverse section of an embryo before lateral flexion of the embryonic plate.

ticulum is homologous with the allantois of lower vertebrates, and the blood vessels which run on each side of it and pass into the body stalk to the placenta are the primitive allantoic blood vessels. That is why the human placenta is termed *chorio-allantoic,* since these primitive allantoic blood vessels vascularize the chorion.

The next change to occur is one of the most important in human development. It involves what is termed *flexion* or *reversal of the head and tail ends* of the embryo; in this process the embryonic plate flexes and approximates its cephalic and caudal extremities ventrally. The transverse axis of rotation of the cephalic region in this flexion is approximately the caudal end of the prochordal plate. Figure 19, showing the embryo in longitudinal section after this flexion has occurred, illustrates the process very clearly when compared with Fig. 17.

At the tail end of the embryo there is another region where ectoderm and endoderm are intimately in contact, called the *cloacal membrane.* This and the prochordal plate represent the sites of the future mouth and anus. The prochordal plate becomes the *buccopharyngeal membrane,* which lies in the depths of the primitive mouth cavity or *stomodaeum,* and the cloacal membrane comes to lie at the base of the primitive anal pit or *proctodaeum.* The intraembryonic mesoderm which forms immediately in front of the protocardiac mesoderm, after flexion of the head end of the embryo, comes to lie caudal to the protocardiac mesoderm which will participate in the development of the heart; this mesoderm, which is the septum transversum, indicates the site of development of the liver and diaphragm.

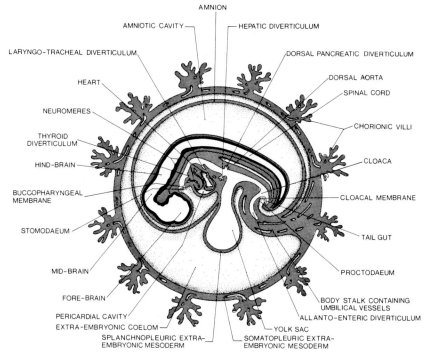

Fig. 19. Diagrammatic representation of a sagittal section through a human embryo after flexion of the head and tail.

Early development of alimentary system

The other very important result of the process of flexion is that the yolk sac is in large part pinched up and incorporated into the body of the embryo so helping to form its alimentary system. The part of the yolk sac which becomes incorporated into the head end of the embryo, i.e. the head fold formed by flexion of its cephalic end, is called the foregut; it lies dorsal to the developing heart, ventral to the developing neural tube, and has the *buccopharyngeal membrane* at its cephalic extremity. Similarly, the portion of the yolk sac included in the tail end of the embryo is called the hindgut. The part of the alimentary system in between these two which remains in wide open communication with the yolk sac is called the midgut, the channel of communication being called the *vitello-intestinal duct* (Figs 20, 21). With further flexion of the embryonic plate this duct becomes narrowed and eventually completely constricted when the umbilicus is formed.

The junction of the foregut and midgut is called the *anterior intestinal portal* and the junction between mid- and hind-gut, the *posterior intestinal portal*. When the blood vascular system begins to develop, the three parts of the embryonic gut are vascularized by separate arteries. These arteries arise from the ventral aspect of the abdominal aorta; the coeliac artery vascularizes the foregut, the superior mesenteric artery the midgut, and the inferior

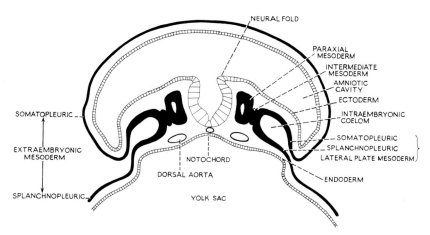

Fig. 20. The appearance of a transverse section of an embryo shown diagrammatically at a time when the intraembryonic coelom has developed and lateral flexion of the embryonic plate is beginning.

mesenteric artery the hindgut. Since certain definite structures develop from each part of the embryonic gut, in the adult only these structures are vascularized by each of the arteries and their respective branches. The foregut forms the adult alimentary canal down to the entry of the common bile duct and all of this part of the gut below the diaphragm is therefore vascularized by branches of the coeliac artery. The midgut forms that part of the alimentary system from the entry of the common bile duct down to the junction of the middle and distal thirds of the transverse colon and therefore only this region of the gut is vascularized by the superior mesenteric artery. The inferior mesenteric artery supplies the remainder of the adult gut (except for the terminal part of the anal canal formed from the proctodaeum (see p. 106)). In the early embryo it is presumed that these territories of arterial distribution are well demarcated, and that there is little or no anastomosis between the arteries. Anastomoses develop in later postnatal life, however.

Intraembryonic mesoderm. Intraembryonic coelom

While the embryo is flexing in a sagittal plane, it also flexes at the lateral margins of the embryonic plate. In order to understand this process it is necessary to comprehend the further development of the intraembryonic

mesoderm, which becomes divided into three parts; most medially the
paraxial mesoderm, alongside the notochord, then the *intermediate
mesoderm,* and most laterally the *lateral plate* mesoderm. The last very soon
shows cavity formation inside it, so splitting the lateral plate mesoderm into
two layers, an upper layer applied to the ectoderm called *somatopleuric*

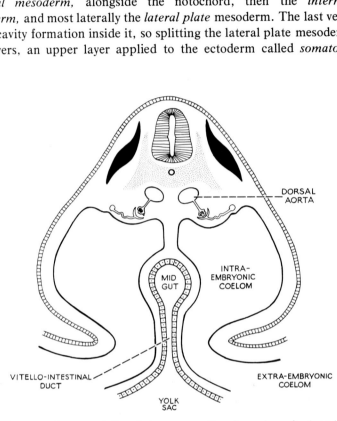

Fig. 21. Diagrammatic representation of a transverse section of an embryo after lateral flexion of
the embryonic plate, so including part of the yolk sac in the body of the embryo to form the
alimentary canal. At this level of section the midgut is seen, still remaining in communication
with the yolk sac by the vitello-intestinal duct.

intraembryonic mesoderm, connected at the edge of the plate with somatopleuric extraembryonic mesoderm, and a lower layer applied to the
endoderm, the *splanchnopleuric intraembryonic mesoderm,* continuous at
the lateral edge of the plate with splanchnopleuric extraembryonic mesoderm.
The cavity that forms in between the two layers is the *intraembryonic coelom*
(Figs 18, 21). The extent of the intraembryonic coelom as seen from the
dorsal aspect of the embryonic disc follows the distribution of lateral plate
mesoderm and crosses the mid-line anteriorly in the protocardiac area, where
it helps to form the pericardial cavity. Because of flexion of the embryo in the
sagittal plane the part of the intraembryonic coelom which is in immediate
communication with the pericardial cavity becomes curved; the process of

flexion of the lateral margins of the embryonic plate also approximates the intraembryonic coelom more caudally situated to its fellow, ventral to the notochord and neural tube, as shown in Figs 20 and 21. This lateral flexion of the embryonic plate similarly constricts the yolk sac, in the transverse plane. The result of these changes is an intraembryonic coelom which is closely related to and surrounds the endodermal gut which has been "taken into" the body of the embryo from the yolk sac.

7

Development of the Somite

The paraxial mesoderm becomes divided into segmentally arranged somites along the length of the embryo, a process called *metamerism*. The tissue of the somite itself soon becomes divided into three parts. The cells of the most medial part, called the *sclerotome,* become condensed and migrate ventrally around the notochord (Fig. 22). They also migrate dorsally to surround the neural tube and join dorsal to it. The sclerotomic tissue differentiates into the vertebrae and intervertebral discs of the vertebral column. Immediately lateral to the sclerotome the cells of the somite become elongated and spindle-shaped and form an oval pale-staining block of tissue when seen in histological section—these cells are grouped together as the myotome, which differentiates into the segmental muscles of the somite in question. The most lateral part of the somite becomes condensed, and forms the *dermatome;* this develops into the dermis or corium of the skin, the ectoderm overlying it forming the epidermis. Any mesoderm of the somite which does not differentiate into muscle, bone or dermis proper will form embryonic connective tissue, which is called *mesenchyme.*

Differentiation of vertebral column

The part of the sclerotome which surrounds the notochord differentiates into the centrum of the vertebra. This condensed mesoderm develops two centres of chondrification; the cartilaginous centrum which results then undergoes endochondral ossification from a single centre. In between the vertebral centra the sclerotome as it surrounds the notochord forms the annulus fibrosus of the intervertebral disc, whereas the notochord in the midst of it becomes modified to form the soft nucleus pulposus by mucoid degeneration of its cells (Peacock, 1951). In the region of the vertebral centrum the notochord completely degenerates and therefore disappears. The migration of the sclerotome dorsally around the neural tube forms the neural arch of the vertebra; when the paired migrations meet each other dorsal to the neural tube they join together to form the neural spine; a centre of chondrification appears in each half of the neural arch. This then joins with the cartilaginous centrum and sends processes laterally to form the transverse process and costal element (see p. 142). Mutch and Walmsley (1956) found that the manner of ossification of the arch closely resembles that in the diaphysis of a long bone. Calcification of the cartilaginous matrix is followed by deposition of bone at the surface immediately beneath the periosteum. Thereafter ossification continues by thickening and extension of this subperiosteal bone,

56

while the calcified cartilage enclosed by it is gradually removed. The ossification is not accomplished by two centres of endochondral ossification, one for each half of the neural arch, as was formerly thought.

The manner in which the sclerotomes serially form the vertebrae and intervertebral discs is rather interesting and important. If a longitudinal section is taken through the back of an embryo it can be seen that the

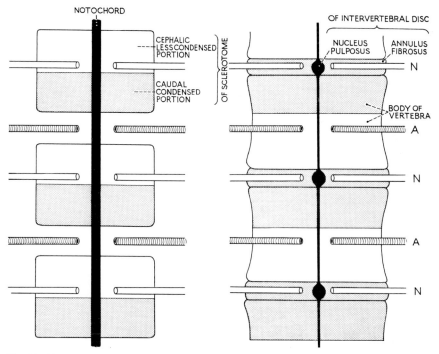

Fig. 22. Diagram showing the formation of the vertebral centra and intervertebral discs from the sclerotomes surrounding the notochord. On the left is the appearance in early development, and on the right the relations of the centra and discs after rearrangement of sclerotomic tissue.

sclerotomes become arranged serially along the length of the notochord; and that the caudal aspect of each sclerotome becomes condensed (Fig. 22) by dense cell aggregation. It becomes demarcated from the cephalic (less condensed) half-sclerotome by the sclerotomic fissure. The cephalic part of the caudal condensed part remains in the middle of the somite (in fact it may move slightly in a cephalic direction (Prader, 1947)) and forms the inter-vertebral disc (Fig. 22), which is therefore segmental in origin. Peacock (1951) has claimed that the intervertebral disc is formed by contributions from both half-sclerotomes, although the major contribution is from the posterior (caudal) half-sclerotome. The caudal part of the caudal (condensed) half-sclerotome joins with the cephalic less condensed part of the immediately caudal sclerotome to form the vertebra, which is therefore intersegmental in origin (Fig. 22). The spinal nerves are strictly segmental and consequently lie in close relationship to the intervertebral discs, which are also segmental in origin, and pass out of the vertebral canal through intervertebral foramina. The arteries which supply the body wall are intersegmental arteries and therefore lie in the adult in close relationship to the vertebrae, which are intersegmental in origin.

It has been claimed (see Strudel, 1955) that the neural tube and notochord in the chick embryo exert a morphogenetic effect on the differentition of vertebrae and their musculature. After birth there are differences in growth of vertebrae in different regions of the vertebral column in rabbits (Tanner and Sawin, 1953) and also between various races of rabbits. This is clear evidence that *shape* in animals is influenced by specific genes.

Development of the skull

Part of the skull develops in close association with somites at the cephalic end of the embryo and therefore can best be considered here. For purposes of convenience in description, the skull during development may be divided into two main parts—the *neurocranium* or brain case, which has a cartilaginous base and a membranous vault, and a *viscerocranium* or splanchnocranium which forms the skeleton of the face, and which is associated with the pharyngeal arches. The viscerocranium also has cartilaginous and membranous parts. The cartilaginous part consists of the cartilages of the pharyngeal arches, structures which are analogous to (see p. 91) the branchial arches of the fish, and which develop from mesodermal cells forming U-shaped swellings lying ventral and lateral to the walls of the pharynx—the membranous part consists of the mesoderm of the pharyngeal arches which condenses around the pharyngeal arch cartilages. The cartilaginous base of the skull undergoes endochondral ossification. The membranous part of the neurocranium develops from the tissue which lies in between the brain and the overlying ectoderm. This is composed of mesoderm intermingled with ectoderm cells derived from the neural crest and is called the *primitive meninx* (Fig. 23; see Sensenig, 1951); it becomes divided into outer and inner layers, the ectomeninx and endomeninx, respectively. The endomeninx again becomes divided into two layers to form the leptomeninges, the pia and arachnoid, while the ectomeninx differentiates on its inner surface into the dura mater and outermost into the *superficial membrane.* It is the latter which undergoes intramembranous ossification in order to form the bones of the skull vault, namely the frontal, the parietals, the membranous supra-occipital and the squamous temporal. The first indication of the development of the cartilaginous base of the skull or chondro-cranium is a chondrification of ectomeninx around the cephalic end of the notochord to form the *parachordal cartilage* (Fig. 23). To this are added more caudally the sclerotomes of the occipital somites. These undergo chondrification and then ossification to form the cartilaginous part of the occipital. The periotic capsule (p. 226) also undergoes chondrification and the otic capsules with their cartilaginous exteriors formed in this way are then added on to the lateral aspects of the parachordal bone to form the petrous parts of the temporal bones. Since the cephalic end of the notochord is at the buccopharyngeal membrane and since the anterior lobe of the pituitary

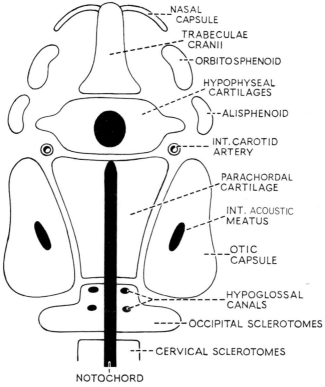

Fig. 23. Diagram of the cartilaginous neurocranium as seen from the dorsal aspect. The base of the skull formed in this way as chondrocranium is seen to be composed of different elements: in the midline these are the parachordal cartilages, hypophysial cartilages and trabeculae cranii. To the lateral aspect of the parachordal cartilages are added the otic capsules.

develops as a diverticulum from the stomodaeum which lies just in front of this membrane, the site of cephalic termination of the notochord in the adult is immediately behind the pituitary gland and consequently immediately behind the sella turcica. It can be seen therefore that a large part of the sphenoid bone including the sella turcica is formed from *hypophysial* or *polar cartilages* which surround the pituitary gland. The part of the base of the skull anterior to the sella turcica is formed from the *trabeculae cranii,* cartilages which fuse together to form the solid bar in front of the sphenoid bone, as shown in Fig. 23. To the lateral aspect of the trabeculae cranii are added cartilages called the *orbitosphenoid,* which forms the lesser wing of the sphenoid bone in the adult, and the *alisphenoid* which forms the greater wing.

Synarthroses

As the base or vault of the skull becomes ossified, centres of ossification appear in the cartilage or membrane concerned. The bones ossified from these centres enlarge and approach each other, but do not fuse for a time, so allowing their further growth in postnatal life. In between the various bones in the base of the skull there is cartilage, and in between those of the vault of the skull, membrane. It can therefore be envisaged how joints between the various skull bones come into being and that these joints are synarthroses. The type of *synarthrosis* in the base of the skull is a *synchondrosis;* for example, the basi-sphenoid and basi-occipital are separated by a plate of cartilage, the occipitosphenoidal synchondrosis. In the vault of the skull, because the bones are separated by membrane forming connective tissue, the bones are therefore separated by joints which are *syndesmoses.* When either a synchondrosis or syndesmosis becomes ossified it forms a *synostosis.*

The cartilaginous components in the viscerocranium do not play a great part in the development of the skull, merely acting as scaffolding, since they consist of the pharyngeal arch cartilages such as Meckel's cartilage and the pterygoquadrate bar (see p. 119) around which mesoderm condenses and undergoes intramembranous ossification to form the maxilla, premaxilla and the mandible.

Overall skull size and the anterior (prechordal) part of the skull base increase six- to sevenfold in linear dimension between the 10th and 40th weeks of fetal life, while dimensions of the parachordal part increase only four- to fivefold; the angles between pre- and para-chordal parts, and between basi-occiput and foramen magnum, consequently become flattened, resulting in increased prominence of the occiput (Ford, 1956), which is very obvious in a newborn child, although a certain amount of the prominence of the occiput in a child born in a vertex delivery (i.e. head first) is caused by *moulding*—overlapping of the skull bones—during parturition.

Development of diarthroses

In the appendicular skeleton, the bones are formed primarily as mesodermal condensations in the limb buds. The latter are produced by localized proliferations of mesoderm in the fore and hind regions of the embryo, forming spade-like extensions which grow in length and then bend at the site of the future elbow and knee. The ectoderm grows uniformly over the surface of the bud (see Tschumi, 1957). The mesodermal condensations chondrify and this hyaline cartilage then undergoes endochondral ossification (see Streeter, 1949; Clark, 1971) to form the limb bones. Ossification of the diaphysis of a long bone occurs first, from a primary centre of ossification which appears about the eighth week of intrauterine life. The pressure epiphyses at each end of the bone are ossified from secondary centres of ossification which appear much later, in postnatal life. The epiphysial cartilage remaining in between the epiphysis and the diaphysis constitutes a primary cartilaginous joint and allows for further growth in length of the bone. The cartilaginous primordia of limb bones also have an overlying separate layer of condensed mesoderm, the perichondrium, which continues over the site of the future joint in between the limb bones. The perichondrium forms the periosteum when ossification has taken place. In between the condensed blocks of mesoderm which form the limb bones is an area of relatively uncondensed mesoderm called the *joint disc* (*interzone*) which is the site of formation of the future joint. In the sutures of the skull, there is a simple transformation of the mesoderm of the joint disc into connective tissue, cartilage or (in later life) bone. In a secondary cartilaginous joint, the joint surfaces are covered by hyaline cartilage, but connected by fibro-cartilage. In addition, in the symphysis pubis there is slight cavitation in the joint disc, but this never becomes lined by synovial membrane. In a *diarthrosis,* which is the most complicated type of joint and the most mobile, the joint disc becomes three-layered. The intermediate third undergoes liquefaction to form the joint cavity, while the other two chondrogenous layers form the articular cartilages. It used to be thought that the cartilage left over the surface of the epiphyses develops into the articular cartilage of the bone, but Haines (1947) has shown quite clearly that the central portion of the latter is formed from the chondrogenous zones of the joint disc. *Synovial mesenchyme,* embryonic connective tissue, migrates into the joint and forms the synovial membrane. It was formerly believed that the perichondrium over the surface of the joint differentiates into the joint capsule, but Haines (1947) has also shown that the capsule is formed quite independently outside the perichondrium. This perichondrium lying inside the capsule (intracapsular perichondrium) is transformed into the more peripheral parts of the articular cartilage. In some joints such as the knee, tcmpoio-mandibular, sternoclavicular, acromio-clavicular and ulno-carpal, there are discs of fibrocartilage inside the joint cavity called *intra-articular menisci.* These and also all intra-capsular structures such as ligaments and tendons are also probably formed from the synovial mesenchyme. The papers of Gardner and Gray (1950), Gray and Gardner (1950 and 1951) and Gray, Gardner and O'Rahilly (1957), which agree in principle with the observations of Haines (1947), should also be consulted. The normal development and maintenance of mobile joints and associated cartilages are dependent on the presence of active musculature.

Development of muscles

The myotome of the somite forms segmental muscles, but muscle tissue also forms in other situations as well. The myotome first of all divides into two separate parts, a dorsal part or *epimere,* and ventral part or *hypomere.* This division of the myotome into two is responsible for three things. First, the site of division itself naturally presents the path of least resistance along which the transverse process of a vertebra can grow. Secondly, since the two parts of the myotome are supplied by nerves, the division of a spinal nerve into dorsal and ventral primary rami also results from this process. The dorsal primary ramus supplies the epimere and the ventral primary ramus the hypomere. Since the hypomere on the whole migrates ventrally into the body wall to form, for example, the intercostal muscles in the thoracic region, the ventral primary ramus migrates with it and therefore becomes more elongated than the dorsal primary ramus. The third and last thing to happen as a result of this division is that the first fascial plane—the lumbar fascia—is formed in the body. The three muscle layers in the thorax, i.e. the intercostals, are really homologous with the three muscle layers in the abdominal wall which are also formed from the hypomere. The ventral ends of the hypomeres bud off along the ventral aspect of the body in every case as a longitudinal column, the rectus column, which can be seen in the cervical region where it forms the infrahyoid muscles, and in the abdomen where it forms the rectus abdominis. In the cervical and lumbar regions the migration of the hypomeres is complicated by the fact that limb buds are present, and a portion of the hypomere may pass into the limb buds in each case to form the muscles of the arm or leg as the case may be. If this is true, migration into the buds probably occurs at an early stage when the myoblasts are relatively un-differentiated and before myotomes as such are recognisable; there is considerable evidence, however, to suggest that limb bud mesoderm is somatopleuric rather than paraxial in origin.

Myotomes also form in the head region of the embryo. Three myotomes develop in front of the otic capsule on each side, the pre-otic myotomes, and these form the orbital muscles. Each myotome is supplied by its own cranial nerve, the third, fourth and sixth in order, and each forms its own group of orbital muscles supplied by its own specific cranial nerve. Gilbert (1957) has described the development of these myotomes and claims that they develop from premandibular mesoderm which is derived from the prochordal plate. Transitory cavities appear in this mesoderm which are homologous with the premandibular head cavities of marsupials, birds, reptiles and elasmo-branchs. Three or four occipital myotomes also develop, but they migrate forwards between the overhanging fore-brain and the bulging pericardium to form the *epipericardial ridge;* this is really composed of mesoderm from the occipital myotomes which travels forwards into the primitive stomodaeum to form the extrinsic and intrinsic muscles of the tongue (see Deuchar, 1958) and becomes supplied by the hypoglossal nerve, the nerve supply to the occipital somites primitively.

Striated voluntary muscle tissue also forms from the pharyngeal arches. Smooth muscle tissue develops from splanchnopleuric intraembryonic mesoderm, which congregates around the alimentary canal to form the muscle coats there, as well as producing the mesenteries and visceral peritoneum. There are two situations in the body, however, where smooth muscle is not formed from mesoderm, but from ectoderm, and these are the iris musculature (p. 221) and the myoepithelial cells of the mammary and sweat glands (pp. 71, 73). There is also one region of the body where the smooth muscle is not derived from either ectoderm or lateral plate mesoderm; it can only be presumed that the intermediate mesoderm which forms the urogenital apparatus also forms the muscular tissue of it.

CLINICAL RELATIONSHIPS

Since the body of each vertebra undergoes chondrification from two centres, if they fail to fuse, the body will be split into two hemivertebrae by an oblique vertical or midline vertical cleft. Double vertebrae can also occur as a result of failure of cephalo-caudal fusion between the two half sclerotomes, a condition called diplospondyly, when the two half vertebrae will lie above one another. Diplospondyly occurs normally in the tails of certain fishes. Occasionally one of the centres of chondrification may fail to appear, in which case there is only one half of a vertebra (hemivertebra). This will obviously lead to a deformity in the vertebral column so that it becomes twisted to the side, a condition called scoliosis. A very common anomaly of vertebral development is that the two halves of the neural arch may fail to join, resulting in spina bifida. It occurs in 1:600-1200 births. In its most minor form, there is no defect in the skin, and the only evidence of its presence is a small dimple often associated with a small tuft of hair; this is called spina bifida occulta. This, like severe cases of spina bifida, tends to occur mostly in the lumbar region of the vertebral column. The condition varies greatly in severity. In the more severe cases the vertebral column defect is associated with a defect in the overlying skin, and the spinal cord and its surrounding membranes are revealed. There may be an associated failure of development of the spinal cord itself. Defects in vertebrae are often accompanied by anomalies of the ribs, which may be absent or fused together.

There may also be a variation in the number of vertebrae in the different regions of the vertebral column. The normal arrangement of 7 cervical, 12 thoracic, 5 lumbar, 5 sacral and 4 coccygeal vertebrae is found in only some 90% of people. The 25th vertebra in 95% of people is the first sacral vertebra. In many other lower primates, however, the 26th vertebra forms S1, but with the evolution of man the 25th undergoes sacralization. The 24th vertebra attempts to do so in some individuals, sometimes even successfully. The 20th vertebra instead of forming L1 may take on the characteristics of T12 as regards the shape of its articular processes and may even bear ribs. Initially the 19th vertebra may not bear ribs. C7, however, frequently is known to develop ribs, and rarely T1 does not develop ribs and becomes more like a cervical vertebra. The development of ribs on the 7th cervical vertebra is of great clinical importance, since such a cervical rib may compress either the great vessels or the brachial plexus as they issue from the neck on their way to the arm. The symptoms of this condition often do not appear until the third decade of life and occur more frequently in women. It may remain symptomless throughout life. It is often possible to feel such a rib at the root of the neck, but its presence may always be revealed by radiography. The symptoms are of three types. Motor disabilities manifest as weakness and perhaps even eventually atrophy of the muscles supplied by C8 and T1, since the cervical rib lies beneath these roots of the brachial plexus. Similar sensory disturbances in the distribution of C8 and T1 may also occur. Vasomotor signs, such as coldness of the hand, and even cyanosis may occur as a result of pressure on the sympathetic nerve fibres in the brachial plexus. The effect of elevating the arm is interesting, since it may relieve the symptoms; depression of the shoulder may have the effect of diminishing or even obliterating the radial pulse.

Occipital defects

The occipital region of the skull represents the fusion of sclerotomes from three occipital somites, and rarely the last of these may assume the form of a cervical vertebra. But in as many as 1% of skulls it is possible to find C1 partly fused with the occipital bone. The centrum of the atlas is made from its own somite (C2) and from the C1 (pro-atlantal) somite. The first cervical nerve, therefore, passes above the atlas. The centrum which develops between the third occipital somite and C1 is a hemicentrum belonging to the pro-atlantal segment and forms the tip of the odontoid process. The C1 and C2 centrum forms the body of the odontoid process, and the C2—C3 centrum forms the centrum of the axis.

Vertebral column curvatures

Until the second month of intrauterine life there is only one curve (anterior concavity) in the vertebral column. At the fourth month it is possible to note that the sacrum is tilted backwards in relationship to the remainder of the vertebral column, so forming the sacro-vertebral angle. As early as the 9th week (Bagnall, Harris and Jones, 1977) the embryo lifts its head and the cervical curve appears. The sacrum itself develops a curve after birth. The lumbar curve in the vertebral column only appears when the child begins to learn to walk. The cervical and thoracic curves and the sacro-vertebral angle are termed primary curves, since they are present in all mammals. The others only appear when there is adaptation to the upright posture. Anomalies in the degree of development of these curves are very common. One such abnormality is kyphosis, an exaggeration of the thoracic backward convexity (hump-back), which may be produced by defective development of both centres of chondrification in the centrum of one or more of the thoracic vertebrae. Lordosis, an exaggeration of the lumbar curvature is very common.

Lumbosacral region

L5 may be fused to S1, probably as a result of lack of separation of the vertebral segments in these vertebrae developmentally. This condition has been shown to be present in King Tutankhamun of XVIIIth dynasty Egypt, and his brother Smenkhkare. The opposite condition, in which L5 is abnormally mobile on S1, is caused by a defect in the pedicles of L5, so that the body of this vertebra slips forward on the sacrum; this disorder is known as spondylolisthesis. Deformities in the articular processes of vertebrae may be related to the presence of a separate centre of ossification, while pedicle defects may result from degenerative changes in the neural arch prior to ossification (Wells, 1963).

Skull defects

Defects in development of the skull may affect either cartilage bone or membrane bones. In achondroplasia there is a defect in the development of cartilage in the epiphysial (growth) plates of long bones and in the cartilaginous base of the skull. An achondroplastic child, therefore, has short limbs, but a normal development of the body and the vault of the skull. Since the nasal bones fuse prematurely the root of the nose is sunken, and the facial skeleton appears depressed below a bulging frontal region of the skull. There is a high palate and lumbar lordosis. Achondroplastic dwarfs usually show perfectly normal mental development; they are often found in circuses and because the condition is always inherited as a Mendelian dominant trait, they may be found associated together in families or colonies. A Bassett hound is an achondroplastic hound. Cleido-cranial dysostosis is a rare inherited condition of partial failure of ossification of membrane bones, and therefore the vault of the skull and clavicles are chiefly affected. The skull fontanelles may fail to close, and because the clavicles do not ossify, the shoulders are abnormally mobile and it may be possible to bring them together across the front of the chest.

In cranioschisis the failure of membrane bones in the skull to ossify is more severe and the vault of the skull is wide open; this is usually associated with anencephaly, in which the brain fails to develop. In craniosynostosis, some of the vault sutures fuse prematurely, so giving rise to an irregularly shaped skull. Thus, if the coronal suture fuses prematurely, the parietal bones continue to grow upwards at the sagittal suture, leading to turricephaly (turret-shaped skull) or scaphocephaly (wedge-shaped skull). When the skull is markedly asymmetrical as a result of irregular premature fusion of certain sutures, this is known as plagiocephaly.

There may be local overgrowth of a part of the skull. If this occurs in the lesser wing of the sphenoid it results in hypertelorism, a condition in which the eyes are abnormally widely separated.

Limb defects

The limbs are subject to many anomalies varying from complete absence of a limb (amelia) to failure of development of only a part (e.g. absent radius or ulna). Partial absence of a limb (ectromelia) may take many forms. In phocomelia only the terminal part of the limb develops; thus the forelimb may be represented only by a hand. Many such deformities occurred as a result of administration of the drug thalidomide to pregnant mothers. Abnormalities of the digits are not uncommon; thus, failure of division of the spade-like extremity of the limb bud leads to syndactyly in which there is some degree of fusion between adjacent toes or fingers. If division of the extremity is more than normally extensive, additional digits (polydactyly) are formed.

During late development there is a gradual eversion of the foot. Even at birth, and always up to the seventh month of fetal life, the feet are inverted. In club foot (talipes equinovarus) the normal process of eversion is arrested. This process of eversion is aided by a shortening of the neck of the talus, the development of the peroneus tertius, and the more rapid growth of tarsal bones in the medial side of the foot.

Skeletal deformities are frequently associated with atresia of the oesophagus, duodenum and anorectal region, further evidence of the fact that disturbances of development commonly affect more than one organ or tissue.

Since muscles develop as a result of splitting of larger muscle masses (e.g. development of extensor muscles of knee, plantar flexors of the ankle joint), migration of muscle tissue (e.g. development of the musculature of the tongue) or combination or fusion of muscles (e.g. development of digastric muscle), many anomalies occur. Thus additional accessory muscles may be found in the arm or leg as a result of excessive fission of embryonic muscular tissue. The peroneus tertius, which is present only in man and occasionally in the gorilla, normally arises as a result of splitting off from the extensor digitorum longus. The palmaris longus is claimed to be an atavistic muscle, and is frequently absent. Other muscles may also fail to develop either wholly or in part, and variations in size (particularly between the sexes) and shape of muscles can occur.

References

Bagnall, K. M., Harris, P. F. and Jones, P. R. M. (1977). A radiographic study of the human fetal spine. *J. Anat.* **123**, 777-782.
Clark, W. E. Le Gros (1971). "The Tissues of the Body" 6th Edn. Clarendon Press, Oxford.
Deuchar, E. M. (1958). Experimental demonstration of tongue muscle origin in chick embryos. *J. Embryol. exp. Morph.* **6**, 527-529.
Ford, E. H. R. (1956). The growth of the foetal skull. *J. Anat.* **90**, 63-72.
Gardner, E. and Gray, D. J. (1950). Prenatal development of the human hip joint. *Am. J. Anat.* **87**, 163-212.
Gilbert, P. W. (1957). The origin and development of human extrinsic ocular muscle. *Contr. Embryol.* **36**, 59-78.

Gray, D. J. and Gardner, E. (1950). Prenatal development of the human knee and superior tibiofibular joints. *Am. J. Anat.* **86,** 235-288.

Gray, D. J. and Gardner, E. (1951). Prenatal development of the human elbow joint. *Am. J. Anat.* **88,** 429-470.

Gray, D. J., Gardner, E. and O'Rahilly, R. (1957). The prenatal development of the skeleton and joints of the human hand. *Am. J. Anat.* **101,** 169-224.

Haines, R. W. (1947). The development of joints. *J. Anat.* **81,** 33-35.

Mutch, J. and Walmsley, R. (1956). The aetiology of cleft vertebral arch in spondylolisthesis. *Lancet* **270,** 74-76.

Peacock, A. (1951). Observations on the prenatal developmental of the intervertebral disc in man. *J. Anat.* **85,** 260-274.

Prader, A. (1947). Die Entwicklung der Zwischenwirbelscheibe beim menschlichen Keimling. *Acta. Anat.* **3,** 115-152.

Sensenig, E. C. (1951). The early development of the meninges of the spinal cord in human embryos. *Contr. Embryol.* **34,** 145-157.

Streeter, G. L. (1949). Developmental horizons in human embryos (fourth issue). A review of the histogenesis of cartilage and bone. *Contr. Embryol.* **33,** 149-167.

Strudel, G. (1955). L'action morphogène du tube nerveux et de la chorde sur la différenciation des vertèbres et des muscles vertébraux chez l'embryon du poulet. *Arch. Anat.* **44,** 209-235.

Tanner, J. M. and Sawin, P. B. (1953). Morphogenetic studies of the rabbit. X1. Genetic differences in the growth of the vertebral column and their relation to growth and development in man. *J. Anat.* **87,** 54-65.

Tschumi, P. A. (1957). The growth of the hindlimb bud of *Xenopus laevis* and its dependence upon the epidermis. *J. Anat.* **91,** 149-172.

Wells, L. H. (1963). Congenital deficiency of the vertebral pedicle. *Anat. Rec.* **145,** 193-196.

8

The Development of Structures from Ectoderm

Epidermal development

The most obvious structure to develop from ectoderm is the epidermis of the skin. The skin fundamentally has two layers, the epidermis and the dermis or corium. The dermis develops from the most peripheral portion of the somite, namely the dermatome; the ectoderm overlying it develops into the epidermis. The epidermis is at first only one cell thick, but soon it forms another layer on its surface called the *periderm,* by a process of mitosis. Mitosis continues from the original basal layer of ectodermal cells to form cells which differentiate into the layers of the adult epidermis which are, from without inwards, stratum corneum, stratum lucidum, stratum granulosum and stratum spinosum. The original layer of ectodermal cells itself forms the stratum basalis (stratum germinativum). When the layers of the epidermis have become established the periderm is shed. Primary and secondary ledge-like penetrations of the stratum basalis into the subjacent dermis form the skin ridges (Hale, 1952).

The stratum basalis continues as an active mitotic layer throughout life, the cells in the superficial strata (termed keratocytes by some authors, since keratin becomes deposited in them) eventually becoming shed at the surface of the stratum corneum. The basal cell proliferation is controlled (in adult skin) by internal secretions (chalones) produced by the differentiating epidermal cells themselves, which inhibit mitosis in stratum basalis cells. The epidermal chalone is tissue specific, but not species specific (Sengel, 1976). There are also other extrinsic humoral or local factors which control epidermal growth. Thus in both embryonic and adult skin the dermis produces a factor which promotes basal cell proliferation.

Hairs

When the skin is two cells thick, it also forms other structures. Thus hairs are formed from localized proliferations of stratum basalis cells scattered over the body surface. Each such initial hair bud grows by multiplication of its cylindrical cells to produce a solid cylindrical downgrowth into the subjacent dermis, oblique to the surface (Fig. 24). The peripheral cells of the downgrowth remain cubical as the hair follicle, and then become organized as the outer root sheath of the hair, while the cells in the middle of the downgrowth become condensed to form the hair shaft and inner root sheath. The base of the hair follicle is invaginated by a small vascular papilla which is derived from the dermis and is therefore mesodermal in origin. The follicle

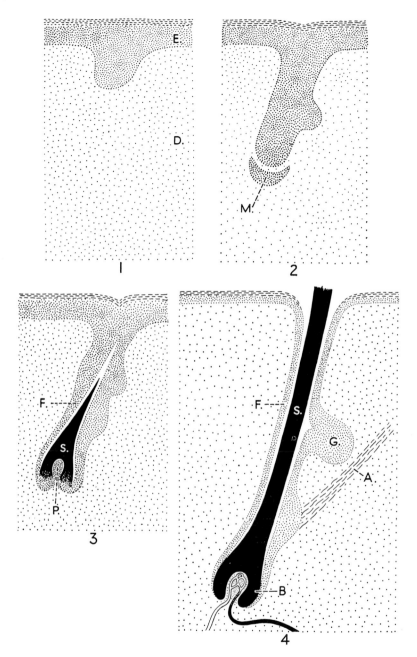

Fig. 24. Stages in development of a hair shown diagrammatically. In 1, a downgrowth from the epidermis (E.) into the subjacent dermis (D.) is first seen. In 2, is shown a condensation of mesoderm (M.) which, in 3, is shown invaginating the base of the hair as a papilla (P.). The epidermal downgrowth becomes resolved into a central shaft (S.) and peripheral follicle (F.). The base of the hair becomes the bulb (B. in 4) and the mesodermal papilla is vascularized by a capillary tuft. An outgrowth from the follicle (seen first in 2) becomes the sebaceous gland (G.). The arrector pili muscle (A.) arises in the dermis from mesoderm derived from dermatome.

base is now termed the *bulb*. There are two sorts of hair formed during development. First of all there is the hair formed during fetal life called the *lanugo* which is shed before birth, and then soon after birth it is replaced by downy hair called *vellus*. This is retained throughout life except where it is replaced by coarse hair in the axilla, and on the pubes, chest and face at puberty.

Hairs are periodically shed and regenerated from the hair follicle in adults. Once the hair has attained its specific length, growth ceases and the follicle becomes quiescent for a while. Alternating morphogenetic, growing and resting phases of the follicle constitute the hair cycle. In man, scalp hair grows at 0·45 mm per day, beard hair having surprisingly the lowest daily growth (0·27 mm).

Nails

Nails are also epidermal derivatives. They are formed slightly later (at the beginning of the 6th month of fetal life) when the stratum lucidum has already differentiated. This latter thickens at the tip of the digit and then migrates on to the dorsum of the distal phalanx, and eventually the stratum corneum degenerates over it except for that which remains at the base of the nail as the cuticle. This migration of the nail has a very important consequence in the cutaneous innervation over the dorsal aspect of the distal phalanx. Because the nail first develops at the tip of the digit it is supplied there by nerves from the palm of the hand and from the sole of the foot. As it migrates it drags with it its nerve of supply so that the sensory innervation over the dorsal aspect of the terminal phalanx is finally provided by palmar or plantar nerves. Finger nails grow faster than toe-nails, and the longer the finger the more rapid the growth. Thus, the middle finger nail grows faster than the thumb-nail (about 100 μm a day).

Sebaceous and sweat glands

Sebaceous glands develop by a proliferation of cells from one side of the hair follicle (Fig. 24). When the.sebaceous glands produce their secretion to oil the hair shaft in adult life, the cells of the gland themselves break down completely. The type of gland in which this occurs is called a *holocrine gland*. There are other glands whose cells only break down in their distal parts in order to produce the secretion. The part of the cell towards the lumen of the gland disintegrates, the nucleus of the cell remaining unaffected; such glands are called *apocrine*. The only glands of this sort are the sweat glands of the axilla (see Charles, 1959) and possibly the perianal region. This may be why the smell of their secretion differs slightly from that of sweat glands elsewhere in the body. All the other normal sweat glands, just like the majority of glands in the body, are *eccrine glands;* in order to produce their secretion they form granules in the cytoplasm which are themselves discharged as the secretion. All the sweat glands are formed in exactly the same way developmentally as a solid epidermal downgrowth into the dermis, the eccrine glands appearing slightly earlier than the apocrine (Montagna, 1956). The base of the downgrowth becomes coiled; the outermost cells of the downgrowth differentiate into the myoepithelial cells which are able to express the secretion of the sweat glands. The lumen of the sweat gland is formed by a breaking down of the cells in the middle of the downgrowth. The fixation of the epidermis to the dermis where sweat gland ducts penetrate serves to direct lateral pressure of growth of the skin inward, so causing the epidermis to corrugate at points marked by the positioning of secondary ridges (Hale, 1952); the sweat glands therefore open at the apices of the papillary ridges.

Mammary glands

The mammary gland is also formed from the epidermis. This develops in all mammals as a thickening of the epidermis producing a ridge called the *mammary ridge* or *mammary line* from the base of the forelimb to the base of the hindlimb bud (see Speert, 1948). Only one localized part, the middle of the cephalic one-third of this ridge, develops into the mammary gland in the human being, but in certain mammals, for example the sow, the mammary glands are formed at intervals along its length.

The thickened epidermis sends down into the subjacent dermis and an underlying fatty pad, 16-24 sprouts which become canalized to form the lactiferous ducts. During the fetal period secondary sprouts and then tertiary sprouts differentiate to produce the ducts and alveoli of the gland; the mesoderm in the dermis congregates just underneath the site of original formation of the downgrowths and elevates the epidermis, so forming the nipple. Insulin is necessary for development of the mammary gland during the fetal period and later (see Anderson, 1974). At birth, whether the sex be male or female, the gland is very rudimentary; but growth and development do not stop then, and since the most important phase of development of the mammary gland takes place after birth, it is necessary to consider it in summary.

Even at birth it is possible for the mammary gland to secrete milk, a phenomenon known as "witch's milk", caused by the passage of hormone across the placenta from the mother into the fetus. This is due to the fact that although the mammary gland may only be at a very rudimentary stage, it is still possible for it to respond to hormones. The male and female mammary glands are fundamentally the same, and when the male is subject to female hormones it is possible for the mammary gland to grow, develop and even secrete milk. This is seen quite commonly nowadays in men above the age of 45 who are treated for carcinoma of the prostate gland with oestrogenic hormones (see p. 177) which may often cure this condition; but after the hormones have been administered for some time they may cause growth of the mammary gland, a condition called gynaecomastia. Androgens secreted in the prepubertal and pubertal male have an inhibitory effect on mammary development. The manner of secretion from the mammary gland, once thought to be apocrine in character, has now been confirmed. Richardson (1947) claimed that only when histological sections of improperly fixed mammary glands are examined is the phenomenon of disintegration of the apex of the secretory cell of this gland visible. In properly fixed histological material this appearance does not occur, and droplets of secretion may be observed being extruded through the luminal border of the secretory cells. Wooding, Peaker and Linzell (1970) have, however, demonstrated the presence of fragments of cell tissue on electron microscopic examination of goat milk, and conclude that they are part of the secretory cells lost in a classical apocrine manner.

Hormonal regulation

The hormonal regulation of the growth of the mammary gland is very important, since approximately 50% of human breast cancers are hormone dependent (Hadfield, 1950). There is no appreciable growth until puberty, when oestrogens and progesterone are secreted. Oestrogens (probably acting synergistically with growth hormone) cause growth of the ducts of the mammary gland, while progesterone (probably acting synergistically with lactogenic hormone) produces growth of the alveoli (Folley, 1955; Crooke, 1958). It has also been stated that the anterior lobe of the pituitary gland regulates growth of the mammary gland by mammogens or mammotrophins since growth of the gland does not occur in the hypophysectomized rat after administration of oestrogen and/or progesterone; but growth does occur in the hypophysectomized rat after other hormones such as deoxycortone are administered or oestrogens or progesterone are rubbed directly into the nipple. These experiments do not exclude an effect of the anterior lobe of the pituitary gland, however, and the answer is probably that all of these factors are concerned. The actual secretion of milk from the mammary gland is quite definitely controlled by the anterior lobe of the pituitary gland. The secretory process can be divided into *lactogenesis,* the initiation of milk secretion, which is produced by lactogenic hormone in conjunction with A.C.T.H., and *galactopoiesis,* a continuation of the secretion once initiated, which is effected by lactogenic hormone in conjunction with another pituitary hormone, probably the growth hormone of the anterior pituitary. Oestrogenic hormones have a profound influence on lactogenesis and galactopoiesis. It has already been shown (p. 23) that small amounts of oestrogen stimulate the anterior pituitary gland while large amounts depress it. This applies to the secretion of milk, so that if small amounts of oestrogen are given milk production is stimulated, whereas if large amounts are administered lactogenesis may cease completely.

The final phenomenon to consider in lactation is the discharge of milk from the mammary gland, the so-called "let-down" of veterinary medicine. This is produced in response to reflex action, since it normally only occurs in response to suckling and quite certainly involves the pituitary gland. It has been shown that the process is probably effected by the secretion of oxytocic hormone of the posterior lobe of the pituitary gland which contracts the myoepithelial cells surrounding the alveoli of the mammary gland and thereby produces ejection of milk from the alveoli along the lactiferous ducts.

Other ectodermal derivatives

Other structures which develop from ectoderm are:
1. The central nervous system including the retina and optic nerve, the lens of the eye and iris musculature.
2. The surface epithelium of the tympanic membrane.
3. The sympathetic nervous system, the peripheral nervous system, the suprarenal medulla, and neurilemmal cells of the peripheral nerves.
4. The epithelium of the mucous membrane of the vestibulum oris and the nasal cavities including the olfactory epithelium.
5. The dental laminae from which will form parts of the teeth.
6. The lower one-third of the anal canal and the terminal part of the male urethra.
7. Rathke's pouch which forms the anterior lobe of the pituitary gland.
8. The sensory epithelium of the vestibulocochlear organ, i.e. the membranous labyrinth.

Teeth

The enamel of teeth therefore develops from ectoderm. This is presaged by a modification of the ectoderm of the oral mucous membrane in the region of the future tooth-bearing portion of the jaws which forms the *dental lamina* in each jaw, a continuous band of thickened ectoderm developed by proliferation of ectoderm cells (Fig. 25). Five proliferations in each maxillary and

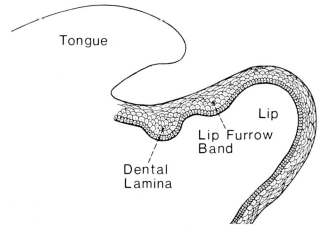

Tongue

Lip

Lip Furrow Band

Dental Lamina

Fig. 25. The earliest developmental change in the formation of a deciduous tooth, showing the dental lamina (D.L.) and underlying mesoderm (M.)

mandibular process (see p. 116) then grow into the subjacent mesoderm and become the *enamel organs* of the deciduous teeth (Fig. 26). The cells in the concavity of the enamel organ become specialized, acquire the capacity of producing enamel and are called *ameloblasts*. The enamel organ becomes concave by a proliferation of mesoderm cells of the dermis to form a *dentine papilla* the cells of which adjacent to the enamel organ differentiate

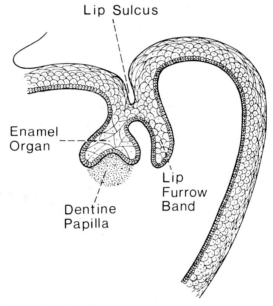

Fig. 26. The proliferation of ectoderm from the dental lamina forming the enamel organ (E.O.) which is growing into the subjacent mesoderm which, in turn, is indenting the enamel organ at one point as the primordium of the dentine papilla (shown in dense stipple).

to form odontoblasts which form the *dentine* of the teeth (Fig. 27). Surrounding the developing tooth the mesoderm cells differentiate to form the *tooth follicle* (Fig. 28), the innermost cells of which differentiate into *cementum* and the outermost layer of cells into the *periodontal membrane*.

An offshoot from the lingual aspect of the neck of the deciduous enamel organ forms the enamel organ of the corresponding permanent tooth (Figs 28-30.

CLINICAL RELATIONSHIPS

Brown fat

The basic pattern of development of the skin and subcutaneous tissue becomes modified in certain regions of the body. Thus, in the interscapular region and around the neck, the human child shows a modification of subcutaneous tissue to form "brown fat". The same modification occurs in the retrosternal and perinephric fat. This fat is similar to the hibernating gland of many mammals in that it is concerned with thermal homeostasis.

The newborn child shivers if it is born into a cold environment. This is a mechanism for increase in oxygen consumption and, therefore, heat production. Shivering is not a prominent feature of cold response, however, and there is another mechanism of nonshivering thermogenesis which involves brown adipose tissue.

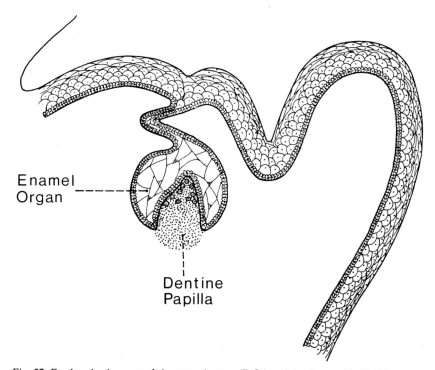

Enamel
Organ

Dentine
Papilla

Fig. 27. Further development of the enamel organ (E.O.) and dentine papilla (D.P.).

When "brown fat" is full of fat it is yellow, but when the fat is depleted it becomes reddish brown in colour because of its high content of mitochondrial cytochrome and the fact that it has a rich blood supply. In low ambient temperatures, the temperature of brown fat remains steady or even rises, although colonic temperature and the temperature of subcutaneous tissue elsewhere, falls. Under conditions of recovery from hypoxia the temperature over brown fat rises more rapidly than elsewhere. Noradrenaline injection also produces similar changes, as a result of pronounced increase in blood flow through the brown fat. More than 65% of extra oxygen utilized during noradrenaline infusion or cold exposure is used by brown fat. Indeed all evidence now suggests that most of the metabolic response to cold occurs in that tissue.

All these considerations are of great importance because of the dire results of inadequate warmth in the newborn child, particularly in premature or small-for-dates babies. The high mortality in premature children in a cold environment may well be related to fat exhaustion in brown adipose tissue.

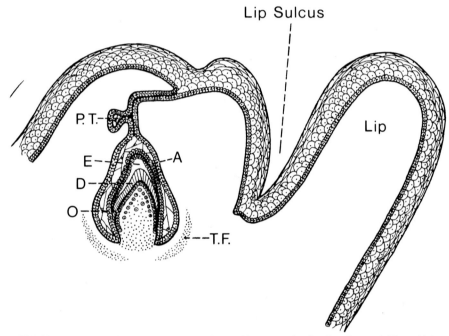

Fig. 28. A later stage in the development of a deciduous tooth, showing the ameloblasts (A.) which have been produced from cells lining the concavity of the enamel organ, and which form enamel (E.) and the dentine (D.), which has developed from odontoblasts (O.) formed from the peripheral cells of the dentine papilla. Mesoderm cells surrounding the developing tooth have differentiated into the tooth follicle (T.F.), and the enamel organ of a permanent tooth (P.T.) has just appeared.

Epidermal tumours

Although dermis has a growth promoting effect on epidermis in embryonic and adult life, the effect is much less in the adult. Dermis associated with epidermal tumours has an effect similar to that in the embryo. It may be assumed, therefore, that growth in epidermal tumours is not dependent entirely either on activity of the stratum basalis, or the activity of chalone-like epidermal inhibitory substances. Keratization of epidermal cells is inhibited by Vitamin A, and sensitivity to excess vitamin A is inversely related to hair production; hairy skin does not react to the vitamin. Hydrocortisone, on the other hand, promotes keratization.

Abnormal hair growth

In man each hair follicle has its own cycling periodicity, but the duration of the cycle in scalp follicles is fairly constant. The morphogenetic and growth phases (anagen) last about three years, the resting phase (telogen) three months. In consequence about 90% adult human scalp follicles are in anagen, 10% in telogen, and less than 1% in catagen (the transitional phase, during which mitosis ceases). Malnutrition causes hairs to be thinner.

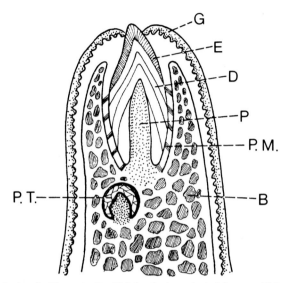

Fig. 29. A developing deciduous tooth which has just penetrated the gum (G.). The roots of the tooth are not yet fully formed. The primordium of the permanent tooth (P.T.), the bone of the mandible (B.), enamel (E.), dentine (D.) and pulp (P.) of the tooth are also shown. The periodontal membrane is indicated lying between the bone and the dentine.

Although androgens bring about the pubertal appearance of hair which grows as a secondary sexual characteristic, in later years they produce a decrease in size of scalp hairs resulting eventually in baldness. Adrenocorticosteroids prolong the telogen phase and shorten the anagen phase, so producing shorter and sparser hairs. Thyroid hormones have the reverse effect and promote hair growth rate (Sengel, 1976).

Hypertrichosis, excessive production of hairs, may be generalized, when it is particularly noticeable on the back of an individual, or may be restricted to small areas. Thus a small tuft of hairs is often associated with spina bifida occulta (p. 63). Alopecia, either total or partial, is due to lack of development of hair follicles.

Abnormal tooth development

Vitamin A is also necessary for the normal development of ameloblasts, and in deficiency of this vitamin the adjacent dentine is also formed irregularly.

In addition to calcium and phosphates, Vitamin D as well as A are essential for the normal functioning of both ameloblasts and odontoblasts. Rubella and syphilis are able to cause malformation during tooth development. The notched incisors (Hutchinsonian teeth) and dome-shaped molars (Moon's molars) of congenital syphilis are well known, but not as common nowadays. Absent or supernumerary teeth are not uncommon and individual teeth may

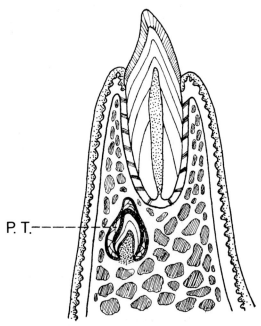

P. T.

Fig. 30. A fully erupted deciduous tooth. The permanent tooth primordium (P.T.) shows further development.

show anomalies of development, such as double crowns or double roots. Imbrication, where one tooth overlaps another, is not uncommon. Often such anomalies have a genetic basis. Anodontia, complete absence of teeth, is very rare and is usually associated with other abnormalities of the skin or its derivatives. The enamel organ has an organizer effect on the dentine papilla and vice versa, so that a defect in one may well be accompanied by some disorder in the other. Since the tendency throughout evolution has been generally to reduce the number of teeth, the presence of additional (fourth) molars has been interpreted as an atavistic tendency, and the imbrication resulting from overcrowding in a dental arch, as evidence of progressive modification.

Abnormal glandular development

It is possible for a mammary gland to develop anywhere along the mammary ridge, from the axilla to the groin. The formation of such accessory mammary glands (polymastia) is relatively uncommon, but the development of accessory nipples (polythelia) occurs in at least 1% of individuals, when they are usually unilateral and occur just below a normal nipple. Amastia (absence of one or both breasts), micromastia and macromastia are all known to occur. Amastia is rare (a total of only some 40 recorded cases in both males and females) and may be unilateral or bilateral. More common is congenital retraction of the nipple, caused by failure of mesodermal elevation of the epidermis at the site of downgrowth of duct sprouts; this may result in breast feeding difficulties.

Sweat glands may be underdeveloped or even absent, when the individual shows anhidrosis, an absence of sweating. This condition may only become noticeable by an individual when he becomes exposed to a hot climate, and finds that he is unable to acclimatize to the high temperature.

Abnormal pigmentation

Pigmentation of skin may be deficient (albinism), or excessive (melanism). The albino even has no pigment in his iris (an ectodermal derivative) so that his iris and his eyes generally appear pink. Total albinism, however, is extremely rare, since traces of pigment can usually be found in the retina by using an ophthalmoscope. After the first few months of postnatal life, skin and eye colour alter little (Harrison, 1961), although there is a sex difference; the skin of white female university students is lighter than that of male students. The individual's pigmentary lability to ultra-violet radiation is the factor concerned in skin colour variation. The distribution of pigmentary differences correlates well with intensity of ultra-violet radiation. Basal-cell carcinoma in human skin may be caused by long exposure to strong sunlight. Since this type of carcinoma is almost unknown in negroes, either a thick stratum corneum, a high melanin concentration or both play an important protective function. Abnormal keratization of the stratum corneum produces a rough, scaly skin (ichthyosis) which may show linear cracks.

Breathnach (1971) in studies of the ultrastructure of prenatal and adult human skin, has shown that the periderm must be regarded as an actively functioning epithelium rather than a purely passive protective layer of cells. It may be concerned with fluid, or other exchange between the amniotic fluid and fetus, and may even have a secretory function.

References
Anderson, R. R. (1974). *In* "Lactation" Vol. 1, Chap. 2 (Eds Lonsen, B. L. and Smith, V. R.) Academic Press, London.
Breathnach, A. S. (1971). "The Ultrastructure of Human Skin" Churchill, London.
Charles, A. (1959). An electron microscopic study of the human axillary apocrine gland. *J. Anat.* **93**, 226-232.
Crooke, A. C. (1958). Treatment of advanced carcinoma of the breast. *Br. med. J.* **ii**, 1425-1428.
Folley, S. J. (1955). Hormones in mammary growth and function. *Br. med. Bull.* **11**, 145-150.
Hadfield, G. (1956). Recent research in physiology of breast applied to mammary cancer. *Br. med. J.* **i**, 1507-1511.
Hale, A. R. (1952). Morphogenesis of volar skin in the human fetus. *Am. J. Anat.* **91**, 147-181.

Harrison, G. A. (1961). Pigmentation. *In* "Genetical Variation in Human Population" Pergamon Press, London.

Montagna, W. (1956). "The Structure and Function of the Skin" Academic Press, New York.

Richardson, K. C. (1947). Some structural features of the mammary tissues. *Br. med. Bull.* **5,** 123-129.

Sengel, P. (1976). "Morphogenesis of Skin" Cambridge University Press.

Speert, H. (1948). The normal and experimental development of the mammary gland of the rhesus monkey, with some pathological correlations. *Contr. Embryol.* **32,** 9-68.

Wooding, F. B. P., Peaker, M. and Linzell, J. L. (1970). Theories of milk secretion: evidence from the electron microscopic examination of milk. *Nature, Lond.* **226,** 762-764.

9

The Foregut

Development of mesenteries

In the development of the liver, a diverticulum grows out from the ventral aspect of the caudal end of the foregut (Fig. 31). This differentiates into the glandular tissue of the liver and is also associated with other diverticula which are to form the gall-bladder and pancreas. Since the foregut develops into that part of the alimentary canal down to the entry of the common bile duct, which is formed from the stem of the hepatic diverticulum, this diverticulum is therefore found at the extreme caudal end of the foregut just before it joins the midgut at the anterior intestinal portal. While flexion of the embryo is proceeding in the sagittal plane, the lateral flexion which is similarly occurring in the transverse plane approximates the two edges of the embryonic plate to each other on the ventral aspect of the embryo, so causing ventral closure of the foregut and hindgut. This process may be appreciated by examining serial sections through the embryo at different levels, as shown diagrammatically in Figs 18, 20 and 21, and it brings the intraembryonic coelom of the two sides into close approximation; the splanchnopleuric intraembryonic mesoderm is also consequently approximated to the endoderm of the roof of the yolk sac. Eventually, as shown in Fig. 21, some of this yolk sac is pinched up into the body of the embryo and covered by the splanchnopleuric intraembryonic mesoderm which therefore forms two structures; first, the mesenteries which suspend the gut in their normal position in the coelom and, second, the muscular and fibrous tissue in the wall of the gut and also peritoneum covering over the gut itself, since the endoderm forms only the epithelium of the mucous membrane. These mesenteries consist of a dorsal mesentery attaching the gut to the dorsal abdominal wall and a ventral mesentery attaching it to the ventral abdominal wall (Fig. 32); but the latter is absent in the region of the midgut which remains in communication with the yolk sac by means of the vitello-intestinal duct. The ventral mesentery of the hindgut soon disappears entirely (Fig. 33). At a later stage the vitello-intestinal duct is constricted and the ventral abdominal wall becomes closed at the umbilicus; if the midgut remains attached to the ventral abdominal wall it does so only abnormally by persistence of the vitello-intestinal duct (p. 107). In the region of the foregut, however, the ventral mesentery persists into adult life; in fact the hepatic diverticulum grows into this mesentery, which is called the *ventral mesogastrium,* since it is attached to the stomach. The somatopleuric intraembryonic mesoderm forms the parietal peritoneum lining the inside of

81

the abdominal wall. The gut caudal to the stomach comes to be supported by a dorsal mesentery but not a ventral mesentery and this reflects the arrangement in quadrupedal animals which only require a dorsal mesentery to suspend the gut from the dorsal abdominal wall.

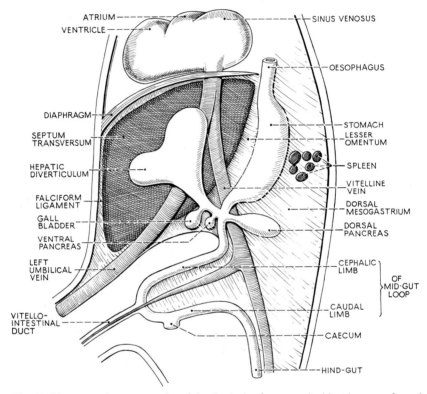

Fig. 31. Diagrammatic representation of the developing foregut and midgut loop seen from the left side showing the diverticula associated with the foregut and the relationship of the hepatic diverticulum to the septum transversum.

Since the hepatic diverticulum grows through the ventral mesogastrium into the septum transversum, two peritoneal ligaments are formed, one passing from the stomach to the liver, the hepatogastric omentum or lesser omentum, the other from the liver and septum transversum to the ventral abdominal wall, the falciform ligament (Figs 31, 34).

The disposition of the intraembryonic coelom at this stage of development is shown in Fig. 35. There is a single unpaired pericardial cavity which is connected to the peritoneal cavity, formed in the manner already indicated, by the parts of the intraembryonic coelom which remain paired and persist as the *pericardio-peritoneal canals* (*channels*). These two canals will form the pleural cavities in the adult.

Development of the stomach

The further development of the foregut can now be considered; it is that part of the primitive gut which is lying dorsal to the embryonic heart and ventral to the neural tube and notochord; its cephalic extremity is indicated by the bucco-pharyngeal membrane and its caudal limit by the anterior intestinal portal. The epithelium of the floor of the foregut (in the chick, for example)

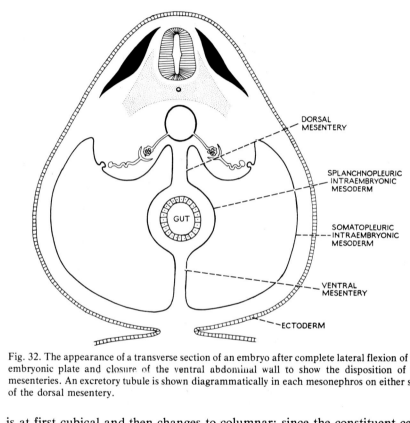

Fig. 32. The appearance of a transverse section of an embryo after complete lateral flexion of the embryonic plate and closure of the ventral abdominal wall to show the disposition of the mesenteries. An excretory tubule is shown diagrammatically in each mesonephros on either side of the dorsal mesentery.

is at first cubical and then changes to columnar; since the constituent cells therefore become narrower, mitotic proliferation is needed to maintain the width of this region but there is no evidence that this is necessary for the morphogenetic movements leading to the ventral closure of the foregut (Bellairs, 1955). A differential dilatation of the foregut develops into the stomach (Fig. 36). The part immediately cephalic to the stomach remains quite short for a long period of time as the oesophagus and the part immediately cephalic to this becomes flattened dorso-ventrally to form the pharynx. The region of the foregut caudal to the stomach forms the first part of the duodenum and the second part of the duodenum down to the entry of the common bile duct.

The stomach, like other parts of the developing gut, is first of all in the sagittal plane of the embryo. Very soon, however, it begins to change its position relative to this plane and the changes that occur can be described in two stages. First, the stomach axis tilts so that the cardiac end of the stomach comes to lie to the left of the sagittal plane and the pyloric end to the

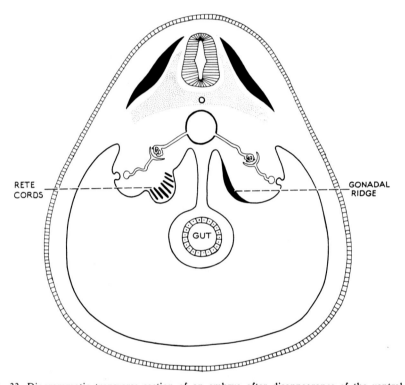

Fig. 33. Diagrammatic transverse section of an embryo after disappearance of the ventral mesentery. The gut is suspended only by a dorsal mesentery, on either side of which there is a thickening of the splanchnopleuric intraembryonic mesoderm on the medial aspect of the mesonephros to form the gonadal ridge (right side of figure) which later becomes larger and develops rete cords (left side of figure).

right (Fig. 37); secondly the stomach rotates around its longitudinal axis so that the dorsal border of the stomach comes to lie inferior (caudal) to the ventral border. The original ventral border of the stomach therefore becomes the lesser curvature and the original dorsal border the greater curvature. Because the dorsal mesogastrium is attached to the greater curvature of the stomach and to the dorsal body wall in the midline, it becomes pulled out and pouched to the left of the median plane as the stomach rotates. The pouch developed in this way, which lies behind (dorsal to) the stomach, is called the *omental bursa* (Figs 46, 47). Kanagasuntheram (1957) claimed that the omental bursa arises by the coalescence of clefts which appear in the splanchnopleuric mesoderm of the dorsal mesogastrium and that lying lateral to the developing stomach; the growth of the bursa and the elongation of the stomach between its relatively fixed cranial and caudal ends produce a flexure of the stomach to the left, so that its original ventral border is now directed to the right. In other words, it is the formation and enlargement of

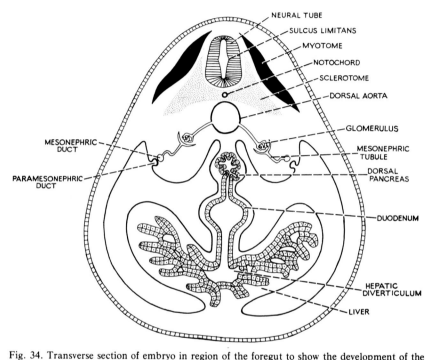

Fig. 34. Transverse section of embryo in region of the foregut to show the development of the hepatic diverticulum from the ventral aspect of the gut, and the dorsal pancreas developing in the dorsal mesentery.

the omental bursa which alters the position of the stomach and not *vice versa*. There is a small diverticulum of the omental bursa just at the entry into this sac which passes cephalically in between the embryonic oesophagus and the right lung bud (Fig. 38); this is the right *pneumato-enteric recess*. Although this structure is very prominent in early development it does not normally form any definite adult structure; it was suggested at one time that it forms a small bursa underneath the heart called the infracardiac bursa (Broman, 1911).

The oesophagus

The oesophagus differentiates from the part of the foregut lying immediately cephalic to the stomach. At first it is very short but as the stomach develops and "descends" to a lower level the oesophagus elongates and in doing so the lumen is almost obliterated, aided by proliferation of its endodermal lining, so that from a very early stage the epithelium is stratified columnar in type (Johns, 1952). At a later stage, however, the lumen becomes larger and as this is accomplished the epithelium of the oesophagus changes to stratified squamous. The endoderm elsewhere in the alimentary canal forms a

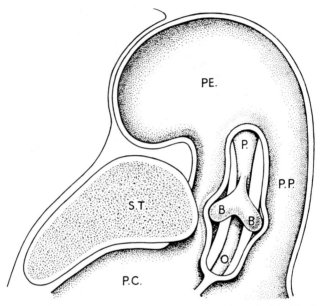

Fig. 35. The appearance of the intraembryonic coelom as seen from the left side after removing the anterior and left lateral walls of the coelomic cavities. The pericardial cavity (PE.) communicates caudally with the two pericardio-peritoneal canals (P.P.) whose medial walls are being invaginated by the bronchial buds (B.). The latter develop from the tracheo-bronchial diverticulum which arises from the floor of the pharynx (P.), which is continuous caudally with the oesophagus (O.). The peritoneal cavity (P.C.) has formed by fusion of the originally bilateral intraembryonic coelom, but the pericardio-peritoneal canals have been prevented from fusing ventrally by the presence of the septum transversum (S.T.).

columnar epithelium and only in the region of the oesophagus does it change to stratified squamous epithelium. There are obvious reasons why the oesophagus should have such an epithelium; it has to withstand trauma and the frequent sudden distension caused by a bolus of food passing down it. This change in histological appearance could be produced in two ways. Thus, a process of *metaplasia* (a change in histological character) in the oesophageal epithelium during widening of the lumen of the oesophagus might occur; there are other regions of the embryonic gut, however, particularly the small intestine, where narrowing or even complete blockage (*atresia*) of the lumen occurs but the gut does not become lined by stratified squamous epithelium.

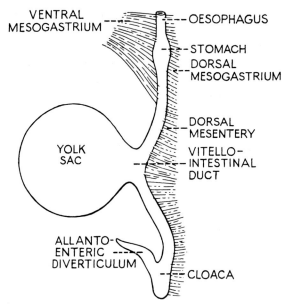

Fig. 36. Developing embryonic alimentary canal viewed from the left side. The midgut is still in wide open connection with the yolk sac.

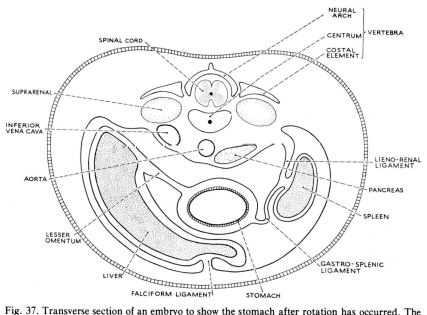

Fig. 37. Transverse section of an embryo to show the stomach after rotation has occurred. The spleen has developed in the dorsal mesogastrium so dividing it into lienorenal and gastrolienal (gastrosplenic) ligaments. The ventral mesogastrium, since the liver has now developed, forms the hepatogastric ligament (lesser omentum) and falciform ligament. The spinal medulla (spinal cord) is assuming its adult form.

For this reason, it has also been hypothesized that the change in character of the epithelium is effected by a migration of cells from the primitive oral cavity. Johns (1952) found that the epithelial transformation occurs first in the middle third of the oesophagus, which would be in favour of its production by metaplasia and Mottet (1970) has recently clearly demonstrated that the transformation to a stratified squamous non-keratinizing

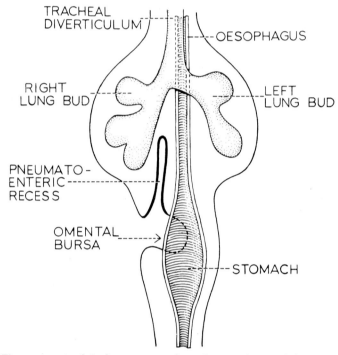

Fig. 38. The appearance of the foregut as seen from the ventral aspect before rotation of the stomach has occurred, showing the pneumato-enteric recess lying between the oesophagus and the right lung bud.

epithelium is by a process of metaplasia, characterized by the interposition of squamous cells between the basal and superficial layers of the embryonic two-layered ciliated columnar epithelium. The superficial mucus-secreting columnar cells subsequently slough off.

Since the stomach rotates to the right, the left and right gastric nerves come to lie anterior (ventral) and posterior (dorsal) to the oesophagus respectively (see also Kanagasuntheram, 1957).

The liver

Immediately caudal to the stomach is a very active region where various diverticula develop. As the hepatic diverticulum grows into the septum transversum (Fig. 34) to form the glandular tissue of the liver, the connective tissue of the liver develops from the tissue of the septum transversum. The branches of the vitelline and umbilical veins running through the septum transversum (Fig. 31) to reach the embryonic heart become broken up by the growing hepatic diverticulum and so form the hepatic sinusoids. As the liver develops it grows more on the right side than the left, so that the right lobe of the liver becomes larger than the left. The rotation of the stomach to the right and the preferential growth of the right lobe of the liver ensures that the hepatogastric ligament should come to lie almost in a coronal plane.

The spleen

While these changes are occurring on the ventral aspect of the stomach, small condensations of mesoderm in the dorsal mesogastrium (Fig. 31) congregate to form the spleen (Fig. 37). This has the important consequence of dividing the dorsal mesogastrium into two mesenteries, one from the stomach to the spleen, the gastrolienal ligament, and the other from the spleen to the kidney, the lieno-renal ligament. Because the spleen forms from independent collections, accessory spleens or *spleniculi* can occur and in the adult spleen there are separate but to a certain extent dependent compartments. Braithwaite and Adams (1957) have shown that each compartment has its own artery and vein. Only under exceptional circumstances, such as congestion in one splenic compartment caused by ligation of its hilar vein, does the spleen become a unified structure and the compartments link up with one another by means of an intersegmental vein. It is also claimed that the spleen has a notch on its anterior border because of this origin from independent collections of mesoderm.

Gall-bladder and pancreas

As shown in Fig. 31, two further diverticula develop from the under aspect of the hepatic diverticulum; one forms the gall-bladder and the cystic duct and the other a diverticulum termed the ventral pancreas. The adult pancreas develops from two diverticula which join each other—the ventral and dorsal pancreatic diverticula. The proximal end of the hepatic diverticulum forms the common bile duct into which opens the cystic duct from the gall-bladder; the duct from the ventral pancreas forms the pancreatic duct in adult life. Both the common bile duct and the ventral pancreas migrate around the right side of the duodenum to come to lie in the mesoduodenum where the duct of the dorsal pancreatic diverticulum joins on to that of the ventral pancreas. It has been suggested (Kanagasuntheram, 1960) that epithelial proliferation in the duodenum contributes in large part to the migration of the biliary opening. The dorsal pancreas forms the neck, body and tail of the pancreas, whereas the ventral pancreatic diverticulum develops into the head and uncinate process; the body and tail of the pancreas come to lie in the lieno-renal ligament dorsal to the stomach (Figs 39, 40). Because the duct of the ventral pancreas forms the adult pancreatic duct and is associated with the development of the common bile duct, these two ducts open together into the second part of the duodenum at the duodenal papilla in adult life. Although normally the duct of the dorsal pancreas joins on to that of the ventral pancreas, occasionally its connection with the duodenum persists as an accessory pancreatic duct.

Since the stomach rotates over to the right and because the head of the pancreas is growing in the mesoduodenum, the duodenum also rotates over to the right and the right layer of the mesoduodenum fuses with the somatopleuric intraembryonic mesoderm of the dorsal abdominal wall, so

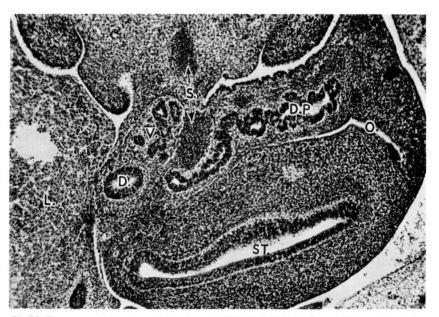

Fig. 39. Transverse section through the stomach (ST.), liver (L.), duodenum (D.) and developing pancreas of a 13 mm human embryo. The ventral pancreas (V.) has come into relation with the dorsal pancreas (D.P.), but is separated from it by the superior mesenteric artery (S.). The omental bursa (O.) lies dorsal to the stomach. (× 69).

that the second part of the duodenum and the pancreas come to lie retroperitoneally. In some animals, namely the pig and the ox, the duct of the dorsal pancreas persists as the normal pancreatic duct, while in others, such as the horse and dog, both ducts and their openings into the duodenum persist. The dorsal duct is sometimes called the duct of Santorini and the ventral pancreatic duct the duct of Wirsung. Both acinar and islet tissue develop from the same diverticula and even in adult life it is possible for acinus cells to become transformed into islet tissue (see, for example, Hughes, 1947; Adams and Harrison, 1953). Because the pancreas develops at the site of junction of fore- and midguts, it becomes vascularized by the arteries supplying both—i.e. branches from both coeliac and superior mesenteric arteries, which eventually anastomose very efficiently (Adams and Harrison, 1953).

The pharynx

Immediately anterior to the oesophagus in the foregut is a region called the pharynx, which becomes flattened dorso-ventrally. This part of the foregut is very prominent in development because it becomes associated with the

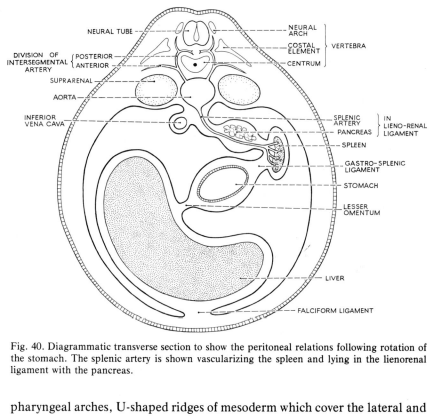

Fig. 40. Diagrammatic transverse section to show the peritoneal relations following rotation of the stomach. The splenic artery is shown vascularizing the spleen and lying in the lienorenal ligament with the pancreas.

pharyngeal arches, U-shaped ridges of mesoderm which cover the lateral and ventral aspects of the walls of the pharynx. These arches are developmentally analogous to, but not serially homologous with, the branchial arches in lower vertebrates such as fish; there are six arches in the human being of which the 5th is rudimentary. The arches lie in relation to the floor and sides of the pharynx and are formed by infiltrations of mesoderm, probably produced from neural crest (see p. 188), between the ectoderm and endoderm in this region. A transverse section of the pharynx shows that the lateral walls are lined by endoderm inside and covered by ectoderm outside (Fig. 41). In between the arches ectoderm and endoderm come into contact at the *closing membranes*. One great difference between the arches in fish and man is that whereas the closing membranes break down in the fish to form the gill slits, they never do so normally in the human being. At the caudal end of the pharynx is a small slit in between the 6th pharyngeal arches. This slit is called the laryngo-tracheal (or tracheo-bronchial) groove and forms a diverticulum which grows downwards ventral to the pharynx (Fig. 41). This is

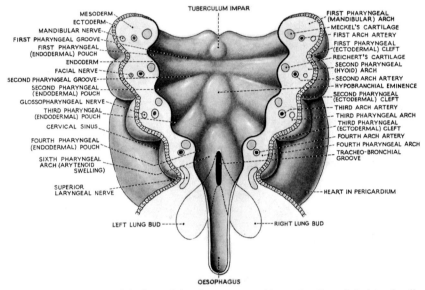

Fig. 41. The appearance of the floor of the pharynx exposed by section through its lateral walls, seen from the dorsal aspect.

the *tracheo-bronchial diverticulum* and soon becomes bifurcate, to form two diverticula which are the *primary bronchial buds* (Fig. 42); these differentiate into the bronchi and their ramifications in each lung. The sixth arches on either side of the opening of this diverticulum into the pharynx become very prominent and form the arytenoid swellings, in which the arytenoid cartilages develop. There is another swelling lying in the floor of the pharynx just in front of the laryngo-tracheal groove called the *hypobranchial eminence;* this develops into the epiglottis, which therefore comes to lie immediately in front of the opening of the larynx. The thyroid cartilages develop from the fourth arch.

The bronchi and lungs

The two primary bronchial buds which are formed as a result of bifurcation of the tracheo-bronchial diverticulum grow in different directions. The right bronchial bud is more in direct line with the trachea and this relationship is maintained into adult life, so that it is much easier for a foreign body to be inhaled by a child into the right bronchus than into the left. The right primary bronchial bud is also larger than the left, since two secondary bronchial buds form from it whereas only one forms from the left (Fig. 38). As a result, there are three bronchi and therefore three lobes of the lung on the right side, but only two bronchi and two lobes of the lung on the left side in adult life. The manner of branching of the primary bronchial bud to give

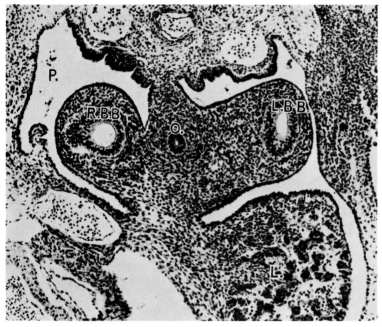

Fig. 42. The developing left (L.B.B.) and right (R.B.B.) bronchial buds of a 7·1 mm human embryo invaginating the medial walls of the pericardio-peritoneal canals (P.). The oesophagus (O.) and liver (L.) are also visible. (× 77).

off secondary bronchial buds is called monopodial (see Hjelmman, 1940). The secondary bronchial buds then branch further and the type of branching is now dichotomous (Fig. 43), in order to form the tertiary bronchi, supplying bronchopulmonary segments, the finer bronchi, bronchioles, the respiratory bronchioles and alveolar ducts. Finally, the terminal branching of the diverticulum produces the aveoli. The structures so formed by this process of branching are derived from the original endodermal diverticulum and only develop into the epithelium of the mucous membrane of the respiratory tract. Because of this, the alveoli are solid and lined by cubical epithelium during embryonic life; the transfer to flattened pavement-like epithelium is accomplished when respiration commences at birth. When the infant breathes air at birth there is distension of the lungs and the epithelium is flattened out to form a continuous unbroken sheet of non-phagocytic alveolar epithelium (Low and Sampaio, 1957). The fetus is now known to display irregular respiratory movements under certain conditions while inside the uterus. It would of necessity breath small quantities of amniotic fluid during this activity, and the inhalation of this fluid may assist the development of air spaces. The fetal lung itself produces an excess of fluid to fill the enlarging alveolar spaces, which may be a necessary morphogenetic factor in their expansion (see Towers, 1959). Surface-active material is also produced in the mature newborn lung as well as in the adult. This surfactant first appears in some animals at the time when the cuboidal epithelium changes to the

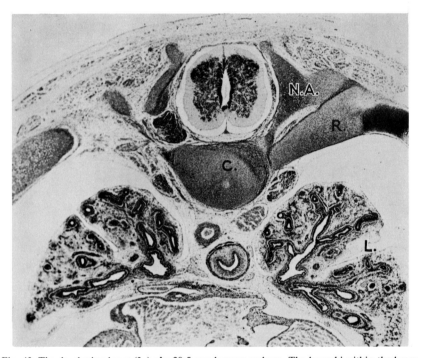

Fig. 43. The developing lungs (L.) of a 28·5 mm human embryo. The bronchi within the lungs can be observed dividing dichotomously and are covered by the splanchnopleuric intraembryonic mesoderm which will form the muscular and fibrous tissue in the walls of the bronchi and connective tissue of the lungs as well as the visceral pleura. The centrum (C.) and neural arch (N.A.) of a vertebra, together with a rib (R.) are also visible. (× 21).

flattened mature type of alveolar cells which are themselves responsible for the discharge of surfactant into the alveoli. Most of the intrapulmonary fluid is expelled through the mouth of the babe at birth by compression of its thorax in the birth passages during delivery. Just as in the gut the splanchnopleuric intraembryonic mesoderm (in this instance, of the pericardio-peritoneal canals, see Fig. 35) covers the structures derived from the endodermal diverticulum and forms the muscle, connective tissue and cartilages of the walls of the trachea (Fig. 44), bronchi and bronchioles and the stroma of the lung in between the alveoli.

CLINICAL RELATIONSHIPS

Occasionally the stomach is known to herniate upwards into the thorax on the right side of the oesophagus through a defect in the diaphragm (the paraoesophageal type of hiatus hernia). Barrett (1954) has suggested that the hernia ascends into a preformed peritoneal sac developed from a persisting

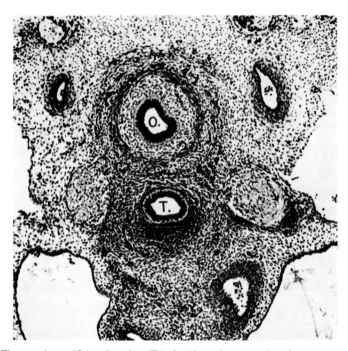

Fig. 44. The oesophagus (O.) and trachea (T.) of a 13 mm human embryo in transverse section. The lining of these two structures, which is clearly visible, developed from foregut endoderm. Splanchnopleuric intraembryonic mesoderm condensing around them can also be seen to be forming the muscle layers and connective tissue. The vagus nerves lie on each side, and lateral to these the anterior cardinal veins. (× 77).

pneumato-enteric recess. The fundus of the stomach may lie on the right side of the abdomen and the pylorus on the left. This is usually associated with complete transposition of the viscera. Congenital diverticula of the stomach are asymptomatic, occur in 0·2% persons and are usually found about 2 cm below the gastro-oesophageal junction.

Gall-bladder anomalies

Congenital defects of the gall-bladder are common enough to require the surgeon to be aware of them during cholecystectomy. Complete agenesia of the gall-bladder is rare in man (0·065-0·042% persons); the rat, horse and elephant normally never develop a gall-bladder. A double gall-bladder occurs in 12% of cats and in some ungulates but is rare in man. A true duplication is associated with two cystic ducts and is usually due to early division or sacculation of the cystic diverticulum. There may be a bilobed or septate condition, or a malformation resulting from a kink at the junction between the body and fundus of the gall-bladder (the so-called phrygian cap deformity) can occur in 2-6% gall-bladders. The gall-bladder can also be found in abnormal situations—under the left lobe of the liver, in between the two layers of peritoneum of the hepatogastric omentum or the falciform ligament, lying transversely under the liver, or even partially or completely imbedded within the liver, which makes cholecystectomy very difficult. It may be posterior to the duodenum or pancreas, or can have a partial or complete mesentery which might permit prolapse (ptosis) of the gall-bladder. Such floating or wandering gall-bladders occur in some 5% of persons and may herniate into the lesser sac or undergo torsion, resulting in gangrene of the gall-bladder.

Defects in liver, spleen and pancreas

The liver or spleen may undergo ptosis owing to abnormally long peritoneal attachments. An increase in lobation of the liver, which occurs normally in lower mammals, is usually found together with duplication of the hepatic ducts and is caused by early division of the hepatic diverticulum. Rarely an elongated tongue of liver (Riedel's lobe) may extend from the right lobe of the liver towards or below the level of the umbilicus, and may be adherent to the hepatic flexure of the colon. Atresia of either the intrahepatic or extrahepatic biliary system may occur once in 20,000-30,000 births; it is a serious anomaly, leading to severe jaundice and death within a year if untreated. This disorder is probably caused by failure of canalization of the ducts which become solid cords as a result of epithelial proliferation at about the fifth week of development. The extrahepatic form may involve only a segment of a duct, a whole duct or the entire biliary system. In the former two instances surgical treatment is possible by removal of the atretic duct and anastomosis of the gall-bladder to the duodenum (cholecystoduodenostomy) or hepatico-choledochostomy in atresia of the common bile duct. There is no treatment (except symptomatic) for intrahepatic biliary atresia and death occurs within four years after birth.

There are common variations in the hepatic ducts such that they unite within the liver (10% individuals), there may be an accessory duct (15·8-24% persons) or duplication of the common hepatic duct. The common hepatic duct may be absent, when the right and left ducts join at the insertion of the cystic duct. In 14-20% persons the cystic duct joins the common bile duct below the level of the first part of the duodenum, and rarely it may enter the duodenum independently. The common bile duct may be duplicated or rarely open ectopically into the first part of the duodenum or stomach.

Splenic anomalies are frequently associated with disturbances of body symmetry. Thus in situs inversus of viscera the spleen is found on the right side, the liver on the left side of the abdomen. Simple splenic agenesia is uncommon, but is found in 3·6% children with congenital cardiac defects. In Kartagener's Syndrome total situs inversus is associated with bronchiectasis and abnormal paranasal sinuses producing chronic sinusitis. Polysplenia, when the spleen is composed of two to nine distinct and relatively equal parts, must be distinguished from accessory spleens, small nodules of splenic tissue which are present in addition to a normal spleen. Since spleniculi occur in 10-31% of the population, this asymptomatic disorder is one of the most frequent anomalies encountered.

The pancreas displays many abnormalities. It has been claimed that persistence of both pancreatic ducts is much commoner than the supposedly normal anatomical arrangement (70% of individuals), and this may be associated with failure of fusion of the parts of the pancreas derived from the two diverticula, and an associated double duct system (10% cases). In 20% persons the accessory duct becomes obliterated before reaching the duodenum. An annular pancreas, which surrounds the second part of the duodenum, the common bile duct or portal vein is a rare anomaly. Accessory pancreases occur in 1% persons and are usually found as nodules of pancreatic tissue which may be found in association with the stomach wall, within the wall of the duodenum or in relation to the spleen. Agenesia, which is very rare, is usually restricted to that part of the pancreas which develops from the dorsal diverticulum.

Oesophageal atresia and fistulae

Persistence of the embryonic condition may result from over-production of epithelial cells in the oesophagus between the 3rd and 5th weeks of embryonic life and consequent oesophageal atresia. Occlusion of the lumen of the duodenum may similarly result from atresia caused by persistence of the epithelial proliferation which normally occurs in the sixth and seventh weeks of embryonic life. Pyloric stenosis may rarely result from such epithelial proliferation, but is usually associated with hypertrophy of the muscular tissue in the region of the pylorus. Oesophageal atresia is often associated with an abnormal communication between the oesophagus and lower end of the trachea (Parish and Cummins, 1958; Smith, 1957). Such fistulous communications are probably occasioned by abnormal adhesion or incomplete separation of the tracheo-bronchial diverticulum from the oesophagus; the atresia in such cases may be so severe as to divide the oesophagus transversely, its upper part ending as a blind sac, the trachea opening into the lower portion. Tracheo-oesophageal fistula occurs once in every 2000 to 5000 live births. Other anomalies, such as absence or atresia of the trachea, complete failure of separation of the trachea and oesophagus and anomalous origin of bronchi are much more uncommon. 50% infants with oesophageal atresia or tracheo-oesophageal fistula have other anomalies, mostly in other parts of the alimentary tract or in the heart. Tracheo-oesophageal fistula is treated by a one-stage intrathoracic operation by ligation of the fistula, repair of the tracheal defect and end-to-end anastomosis of the upper and lower segments of the oesophagus.

The oesophagus may not elongate sufficiently from its embryonic condition, so resulting in a congenitally short oesophagus; this, in turn, is usually associated with some degree of "thoracic stomach". Such cases are rare and may be distinguished from hiatus hernia by the fact that the herniated portion of the stomach in the latter condition is vascularized by the left gastric artery and is accompanied by a peritoneal sac.

Achalasia of the cardia, a condition in which muscle fibres at the oesophago-gastric junction are unable to relax, is probably caused by a defect in the development of the myenteric plexus in this region. It leads to a difficulty in swallowing and regurgitation of food, and can often be cured by dilating the lower end of the oesophagus with a bougie.

Bronchial anomalies

The failure of the upper (apical; eparterial) bronchus to develop as an independent structure with its own lobe on the left side has been variously interpreted by different authorities. The result of diminished pulmonary expansion consequent upon the pressure of the heart, and relative descent of the aortic arch together with the heart, are two widely held theories. Others claim that the apical bronchus of the right upper lobe is a tertiary bronchus which has migrated cephalically, assumed dominance and organized the development of a new lobe around itself. Nevertheless an eparterial bronchus and even an upper lobe may develop abnormally on the left side, and evidence of cephalic migration of the right apical bronchus is provided by the fact that this bronchus arises from the trachea in some ungulates and may occasionally do so in man. These features are extremely important to remember in lobectomy operations.

Unilateral agenesis of a lung is uncommon (1 in 15,000 persons) and is occasioned by developmental imbalance between the two lung buds. If the right lung is absent, the left is frequently tri-lobed. 50% of cases of pulmonary agenesis possess other anomalies.

Cysts can be found in the lungs of some infants and children (0·04-0·06% children) and may be congenital in origin. They may be bronchiolar or alveolar in origin, single or multiple.

Hyaline membrane disease

Surfactant is absent from the lungs of human infants dying from the respiratory distress syndrome (hyaline membrane disease). As a result, it is impossible to overcome surface-tension in the alveoli when the lungs are inflated at birth. The alveoli, therefore, cannot ventilate adequately and the child suffers considerable hypoxaemia. This is sufficient to result in 30% of deaths of all newborn children and as much as 70% of deaths in premature children.

References

Adams, D. J. and Harrison, R. G. (1953). The vascularization of the rat pancreas and the effect of ischaemia on the islets of Langerhans. *J. Anat.* **87**, 257-267.

Barrett, N. R. (1954). Hiatus hernia. *Br. J. Surg.* **42**, 231-244.

Bellairs, R. (1955). Studies on the development of the foregut in the chick. III. The role of mitosis. *J. Embryol. exp. Morph.* **3**, 242.

Braithwaite, J. L. and Adams, D. J. (1957). The venous drainage of the rat spleen. *J. Anat.* **91**, 352-359.

Broman, I. (1911). "Normale und Abnorme Entwicklung des Menschen" p. 367. Bergmann, Wiesbaden.

Hjelmman, G. (1940). Zur kenntnis der embryonalentwicklung der lungen des Rindes. *Morph Jb.* **84**, 491-540.

Hughes, H. (1947). Cyclical changes in the islets of Langerhans in the rat pancreas. *J. Anat.* **81**, 82-92.

Johns, B. A. E. (1952). Developmental changes in the oesophageal epithelium in man. *J. Anat.* **86**, 431-442.

Kanagasuntheram, R. (1957). Development of the human lesser sac. *J. Anat.* **91**, 188-206.

Kanagasuntheram, R. (1960). Some observations on the development of the human duodenum. *J. Anat.* **94**, 231-240.

Low, F. N. and Sampaio, M. M. (1957). The pulmonary alveolar epithelium as an entodermal derivative. *Anat. Rec.* **127**, 51-64.

Mottet, N. K. (1970). Mucin biosynthesis by chick and human oesophagus during autogenetic metaplasia. *J. Anat.* **107**, 49-66.

Parish, C. and Cummins, C. F. A. (1958). Oesophageal atresia. Experience in 17 cases, with notes on operative technique. *Brit. med. J.* **ii**, 1140-1144.

Smith, E. I. (1957). The early development of the trachea and oesophagus in relation to atresia of the oesophagus and tracheoesophageal fistula. *Contr. Embryol.* **36**, 41-60.

Towers, B. (1959). Amniotic fluid and the foetal lung. *Nature, Lond.* **183**, 1140-1141.

10

Midgut and Hindgut

The midgut loop

The midgut is that part of the alimentary canal in wide open communication with the yolk sac and is continuous caudally with the hindgut into which opens the allanto-enteric diverticulum. The primitive alimentary canal in the embryo is first of all in the axial region of the embryo and stays there for some time. The midgut at first has a mesentery no longer than that of the foregut and hindgut but later it acquires a longer dorsal mesentery by forming the midgut loop which comes to lie in a part of the extraembryonic coelom called the umbilical sac, in the region of the future umbilicus. In other words, the midgut loop comes to lie outside the intraembryonic coelom of the embryo. The apex of the midgut loop is continuous with the vitello-intestinal duct and the yolk sac (Fig. 45). The midgut loop therefore has two limbs, the cephalic lying cephalic to the vitello-intestinal duct which develops into the first 18 to 20 feet of the small intestine, and the caudal limb which will form approximately the last 2 feet of the small intestine, ascending colon and the proximal two-thirds of the transverse colon. The midgut loop in the extraembryonic coelom then rotates through 90° so that the cephalic limb is on the right side of the caudal limb. The cephalic limb soon increases in length since it is to form most of the small intestine; the umbilical sac cannot accommodate it and therefore it must return to the abdominal cavity. As the cephalic limb returns it does so on the right side of the hindgut and its mesentery. In consequence, the hindgut, which develops into the descending and sigmoid (pelvic) colon and cloaca, is pushed over to the left side of the abdomen. The cephalic limb of the midgut loop tends to fill up the abdominal cavity and when the caudal limb returns to the coelom it can only come to lie above the small intestine already formed by the cephalic limb of the midgut loop, since the termination of the caudal limb is still attached to the hindgut on the left side of the abdomen (Fig. 46).

While the caudal limb is in the umbilical sac, it develops a swelling which becomes the caecum; this swelling is said to hold the caudal limb inside the sac and delay its return to the peritoneal cavity until after the cephalic limb (see Snyder and Chaffin, 1952). At about this time also the liver is diminishing in size as a result of a decrease in the relative number of hepatic cells (see Dick, 1956); a resultant increased negative intra-abdominal pressure (see Wyburn, 1939) and also probably more room inside the abdominal cavity, facilitate the return of the midgut loop. Kanagasuntheram (1960) has suggested that the return of the midgut loop is due to contraction of the longitudinal musculature of the duodenum and proximal jejunum. The vitello-intestinal duct and yolk sac undergo atrophy and completely disappear.

When the caudal limb of the midgut loop returns, the caecum comes to lie in a position just below the liver and while here the appendix is differentiated by a lag in growth of part of the caecum. Later the caecum with the appendix

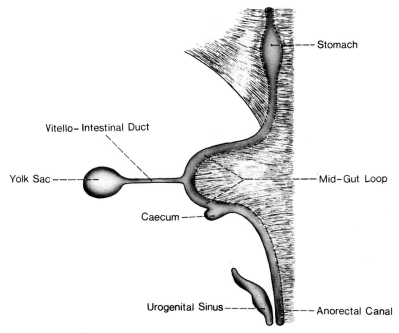

Fig. 45. The appearance of the midgut loop as seen from the left side at a later stage than Fig. 36, after the vitello-intestinal duct has become constricted.

descends to its normal adult position (Fig. 47). Because the cranial limb of the midgut loop comes to lie on the right side but also slightly below the caudal limb, the majority of the small intestine will lie below the point of origin of the superior mesenteric vessels (Fig. 48).

The hindgut

The hindgut is continuous with the caudal limb of the midgut loop and terminates in the cloaca which possesses the diverticulum called the allanto-enteric diverticulum; caudal to the cloaca is a small portion of the embryonic gut called the tail gut. The endodermal cloaca is in close contact with the ectoderm with no intervening mesoderm at the *cloacal membrane*. When this membrane later breaks down the gut communicates with the exterior but although the fetus swallows liquor amnii containing mucus and keratin squames from its own skin, they are not normally defaecated until after birth because the expulsive action of the rectum and anus is absent although the small intestine has some peristaltic activity. Within 24 hours after birth, motions coloured with bilirubin and called *meconium* are passed by the infant.

Dorsal to the tail gut the notochord ends in a mass of undifferentiated mesodermal tissue which represents the remains of the primitive streak (Fig.

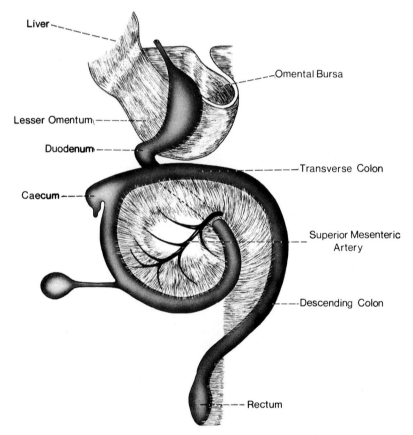

Fig. 46. The disposition of the midgut loop following its return to the coelom as seen from the ventral aspect, showing its relation to other parts of the embryonic alimentary canal.

49). This region undergoes atrophy, and is shed from the body. Before the primitive streak is lost in this way, it produces mesoderm which migrates around on either side of the cloaca and comes to lie ventral to the cloaca in the region between the cloacal membrane and the allanto-enteric diverticulum (Figs 50, 51). Since the apex of the latter lies in the umbilicus this mesoderm must form the infraumbilical region of the body wall; it may be contributed to by extraembryonic mesoderm and congregates at the cephalic end of the cloacal membrane. It cannot infiltrate between the ectoderm and endoderm of this membrane, however, and by pushing on its cephalic extremity may cause it to rotate so that it comes to face in a caudal direction as shown in Fig. 51. The congregation of mesoderm itself raises up a tubercle called the *genital tubercle,* which differentiates into the clitoris in the female and the glans penis in the male.

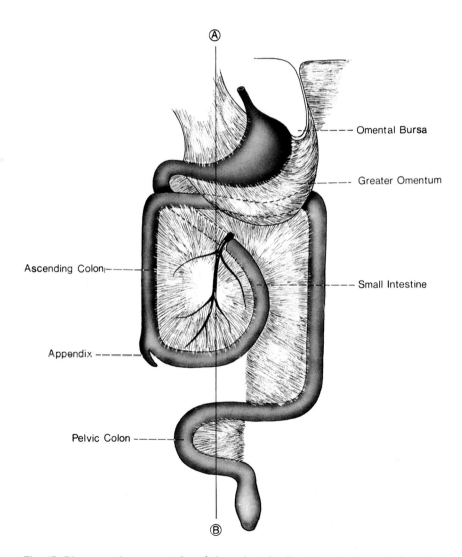

Fig. 47. Diagrammatic representation of the embryonic alimentary canal as seen from the ventral aspect following descent of the caecum to its adult position.

Development of the cloaca

A septum forms in the angle between the allanto-enteric diverticulum and the caudal end of the hindgut. This septum, which is composed of mesoderm, is the *urorectal septum* and divides the cloaca into two parts, the *urogenital sinus* ventrally and the *anorectal canal* dorsally (see Politzer, 1931). It also divides the cloacal membrane into two parts, the urogenital

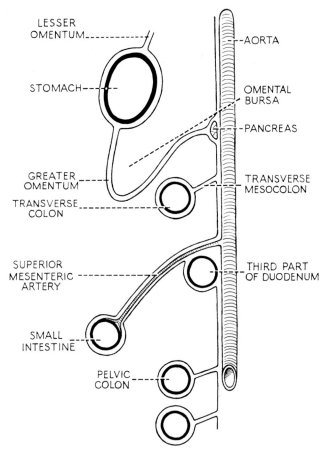

Fig. 48. The appearance of a sagittal section of the embryonic alimentary canal along line **AB** in Fig. 47, seen from the left side.

membrane ventrally and the anal membrane dorsally. This division of the cloaca is also aided by an increased growth in the caudal part of the anorectal canal (Forsberg, 1961). The anorectal canal forms the whole of the rectum and the upper two-thirds (the upper 2·5 cm) of the adult anal canal. The lower one-third of the anal canal is formed by the sinking in of the anal membrane to form a pit called the *proctodaeum,* and this is accomplished by

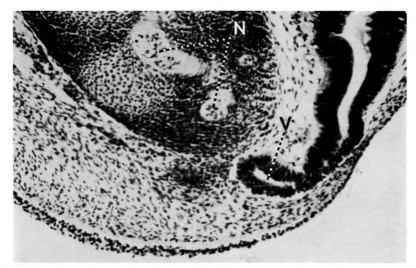

Fig. 49. Longitudinal section through the tail of a 17 mm human embryo to show the notochord (N.) ending in a mass of undifferentiated tissue which probably represents the remains of the primitive streak. The ventriculus terminalis (v. see p. 192) is also shown. (× 690).

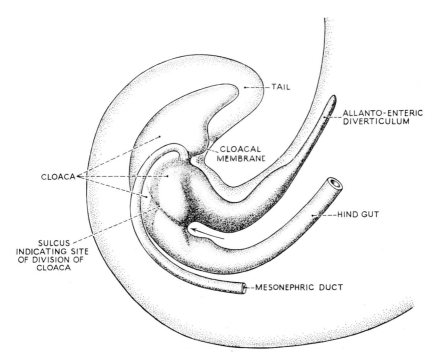

Fig. 50. The appearance of the cloaca in early development as seen from the left side. The arrow indicates the position and direction of growth of the urorectal septum.

the anal membrane being surrounded by the mesoderm already described as being produced by primitive streak, so elevating the ectoderm around the anal membrane which consequently becomes depressed below the surface.

The anal canal therefore has a double origin consequent upon its development. The upper two-thirds, developed from the anorectal canal, is lined by endoderm and has a columnar epithelium; the mucous membrane of

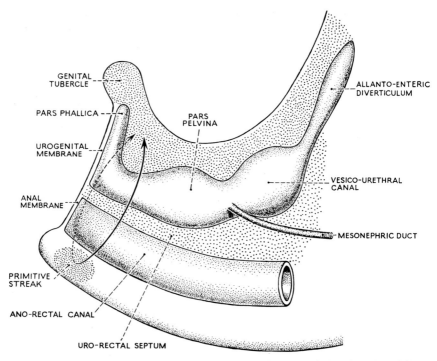

Fig. 51. Diagrammatic appearance of the tail region, seen from the left side, following division of the cloaca into a ventral urogenital sinus and dorsal anorectal canal. The arrows show the direction of migration of mesoderm from the primitive streak towards the ventral aspect of the embryo to produce the genital tubercle and mesoderm of the infra-umbilical region of the body wall.

this part of the anal canal has mucous glands. The lower one-third of the anal canal, however, is lined by ectoderm which forms a stratified squamous epithelium and in it there are sebaceous glands and modified sweat glands. The upper two-thirds for the same reason becomes vascularized by the artery of the hindgut, namely a terminal branch of the inferior mesenteric artery, the superior rectal artery, whereas the lower one-third of the anal canal is supplied by systemic arteries, namely the middle and inferior rectal arteries, branches of the internal iliac and pudendal arteries. The corresponding veins drain in a similar fashion.

CLINICAL RELATIONSHIPS

Exomphalos

If the midgut loop remains in the umbilical sac and does not return to the abdominal cavity, the baby is born with its intestines protruding from the umbilicus in a sac, an anomaly occurring once in 1860-3200 births. In some 50% of cases of *exomphalos,* as the condition is called, both small and large intestine and a variable proportion of the liver may be present in the sac. The wall of the sac is three layered, consisting of peritoneum, extraembryonic mesoderm which has formed Wharton's jelly, and amnion. The umbilical cord is attached to the apex of the sac in exomphalos minor, or to its inferior aspect in severe cases. In such exomphalos major, which requires surgical operation within the first few hours of life to obviate the sac bursting, it is often very difficult to replace and accommodate the contents of the sac in an abdominal cavity that has never housed them, so that a two stage closure of the abdominal wall is necessary. Exomphalos should be distinguished from congenital umbilical hernia which is a rare condition in which a small exomphalos has been closed over by skin before birth, and no umbilical sac is visible. The umbilical hernia of infants and children, and certainly that occurring in adults may be para-umbilical in that it emerges through the linea alba above or below the umbilicus.

Meckel's diverticulum

A persistence of the vitello-intestinal duct in 2% of persons results in a *Meckel's diverticulum.* Such a diverticulum may or may not be attached at its apex to the umbilicus, and arises from the gut at a point which represents the apex of the midgut loop in the embryo. Thus it is to be found arising from the ileum approximately 40-60 cm from the ileocaecal junction—although, in describing measurements of the adult small intestine it should be remembered that variations of as much as 100% in its total length can occur (Underhill, 1955). Rarely an inguinal hernia may contain a Meckel's diverticulum, when it is called Littre's hernia (Meyerowitz, 1958), and such a diverticulum may be found in the umbilical sac of exomphalos. The diverticulum in the adult varies considerably in length (1-60 cm) and arises from the antimesenteric border of the ileum. A Meckel's diverticulum may remain symptomless ("silent") throughout life, but may announce its presence in several ways. Thus, if it remains attached to the umbilicus (25% cases), it forms a bar in the peritoneal cavity, particularly if the diverticulum becomes obliterated to form a band, around which intestine may become obstructed or even strangulated. Heterotopic gastric mucosa can occur in a Meckel's diverticulum, which may undergo ulceration, and the resulting ulcer may even perforate. If an attached diverticulum perforates through to the surface, an *umbilical fistula* results, with the appearance of faeces at the umbilicus.

Symmetry reversal

The distal limb of the midgut loop may return to the abdominal cavity incorrectly, so that while the small intestine lies predominantly on the right side of the abdomen, the ascending colon is found on the left. Arrest of the normal process of rotation of the midgut loop (0·5% persons), or complete rotation, can lead to the most bizarre relationships in the adult (Wilson, 1964), particularly in the relative positions of the pancreas and duodenum. Reversed torsion of the loop may result in the transverse colon lying posterior to the duodenum. There may be complete transposition of the alimentary tract, the relationships being a mirror image of the normal anatomy—this occurs in the condition known as situs inversus.

Such transposition of viscera has been claimed to be part of a symmetry reversal which may be expressed in some individuals in very minor form, such as left handedness or even a counter-clockwise hair whorl on the head.

The subhepatic position of the caecum may be maintained into adult life. The abdominal surgeon must be aware of these abnormalities when encountering variations from the normal during his operations.

Imperforate anus

If the anal membrane fails to break down, an imperforate anus may result, and is of varying degrees of severity. There may be a persistence of the whole membrane, or it may rupture incompletely, leading to anal stricture. In more severe cases the anal canal also appears to undergo atresia as a result of proliferation of its lining epithelium; the rectum, therefore, ends blindly at a variable distance from the external anal sphincter. Anorectal defects occur once in 3500 births. In about 50% of severe cases of imperforate anus, there is a fistula into the bladder or urethra. This condition of rectovesical or rectourethral fistula is caused by failure of the urorectal septum to develop properly; an early symptom of this disorder is the presence of gas in the urine. In the female, a rectovaginal fistula occurs. Imperforate anus is associated with other congenital anomalies, particularly of the excretory system, in 70% cases. In severe cases a colostomy may have to be performed until the local condition can be treated surgically at one year of age. In mild cases, particularly without a fistula, an ano-proctoplasty can be undertaken immediately.

Persistent tail

The tail of the embryo reaches its maximum size at the end of the fifth week of embryonic life, when it is about one sixth of the length of the embryo. It normally disappears during the next month, mainly because the coccyx, which is all that persists, recedes to a higher level. Externally the only postnatal evidence of the tail is the postanal fovea or pit. Abnormally the tail may persist as a fleshy appendage as long as 7 cm; it may rarely contain degenerate caudal vertebrae. The persistence and unregulated activity of primitive streak cells in a tail rudiment has been imputed in the development of a sacrococcygeal tumour, a rare teratoma containing almost any sort of tissue and present at birth. These tumours may be so large as to cause difficulties in childbirth and in 20% cases the babe is stillborn.

Atresia

Narrowing (stenosis) or complete blockage (atresia) of some part of the intestines leads to intestinal obstruction. Atresia, which occurs once in 1500 births, may be due to failure of recanalization after epithelial occlusion, and is most common in the duodenum; it is rare in the colon. Stenosis is much rarer and occurs almost entirely in the duodenum; it is usually associated with annular pancreas. The treatment of atresia is by surgical resection of the affected bowel with end-to-end or side-to-side anastomosis of the remaining healthy intestine.

Developmental defects in the musculature of the intestine can lead to diverticula. These are most common in the duodenum (2·7% persons) and mostly (75%) in the descending (second) part, and are usually asymptomatic. Diverticula also occur in the jejunum and ileum, but their presence in the colon (diverticulosis) is largely restricted to the descending colon in persons of mature and increasing age; they are very rare in persons under 30 years of age, which suggests that they are not of congenital origin.

The transverse (third) part of the duodenum may be compressed by an abnormal superior mesenteric artery. The resultant superior mesenteric artery syndrome is occasioned by compression of the duodenum by the artery against the aorta and L2/3 vertebrae, so causing an acute, chronic or intermittent intestinal obstruction.

References

Dick, D. A. T. (1956). Growth and function in the foetal liver. *J. Embryol. exp. Morph.* **4**, 97-109.

Forsberg, J.-G. (1961). On the development of the cloaca and the perineum and the formation of the urethral plate in female rat embryos. *J. Anat.* **95**, 423-436.

Kanagasuntheram, R. (1960). Some observations on the development of the human duodenum. *J. Anat.* **94**, 231-240.

Meyerowitz, B. R. (1958). Littre's hernia. *Brit. med. J.* **i**, 1154-1156.

Politzer, G. (1931). Uber die entwicklung des dammes beim menschen. *Z. Anat. EntwGesch.* **95**, 734-768.

Snyder, W. H. and Chaffin, L. (1952). An intermediate stage in the return of the intestines from the umbilical cord (Embryo 37mm). *Anat. Rec.* **113**, 451-457.

Underhill, B. M. L. (1955). Intestinal length in man. *Brit. med. J.* **ii**, 1243-1246.

Wilson, P. M. (1964). Unusual duodeno-pancreatic relationships associated with incomplete rotation of mid-gut loop. *Anat. Rec.* **149**, 397-404.

Wyburn, G. M. (1939). The formation of the umbilical cord and the umbilical region of the anterior abdominal wall. *J. Anat.* **73**, 289.

11

Diaphragm and Pleural Cavities

Development of pleural sacs

Due to flexion of the lateral margins of the embryonic plate, the two intraembryonic coeloms are approximated on the ventral aspect of the embryo and fuse together in the region of the peritoneal cavity. This also occurs in the formation of the pericardial cavity, in addition to the development of part of it in the protocardiac area immediately cephalic to the prochordal plate, before it is carried on to the ventral aspect of the embryo by the flexion of its head end. The unpaired pericardial cavity on the ventral aspect of the foregut communicates with the unpaired peritoneal cavity more caudally situated by the still paired intraembryonic coeloms in between the two, as shown in Fig. 35; these two channels of communication are called the *pericardio-peritoneal canals.* Figure 35 demonstrates that the septum transversum, which is a large block of mesoderm lying immediately caudal to the heart, prevents the pericardio-peritoneal canals from approximating to one another and fusing on the ventral aspect of the embryo, since it is lying in the position where they would be expected to fuse. It has already been mentioned that the caudal aspect of this septum is the site of growth of the hepatic diverticulum. The cephalic part of the septum transversum is just as important, because it develops into a large portion of the diaphragm.

Each pericardio-peritoneal canal develops into a pleural cavity and, in order that it can be shut off from the pericardial cavity, a membrane called the *pericardio-pleural* membrane closes the opening from the pericardial cavity into the pericardio-peritoneal canal. A similar membrane, namely the *pleuro-peritoneal membrane,* develops at the site of communication between each pericardio-peritoneal canal and the peritoneal cavity. The pericardio-pleural membrane is formed in association with the common cardinal vein, or duct of Cuvier, which lies immediately lateral to the pericardio-pleural openings; as the heart "descends" in development, this vein becomes more obliquely orientated and invaginates the lateral wall of the pericardio-pleural opening, so raising up the fold which becomes the pericardio-pleural membrane (Fig. 52). The pericardio-pleural membranes later contact each other, fuse to form fibrous pericardium and shut off the pericardio-pleural openings (Fig. 53). The pleuro-peritoneal membrane, probably formed by delamination of the body wall, closes the pleuro-peritoneal opening.

Contributions to diaphragm

The septum transversum is ideally situated to form a large portion of the diaphragm, since it lies immediately caudal to the pericardial cavity and on the same horizontal level as the pleuro-peritoneal openings. The pleuro-peritoneal membranes also form a portion of the diaphragm (Fig. 54), lying dorso-lateral to the septum transversum. The bronchial (lung) buds invaginate the medial wall of the pericardio-peritoneal canals, and so become covered by the splanchnopleuric intraembryonic mesoderm which forms this

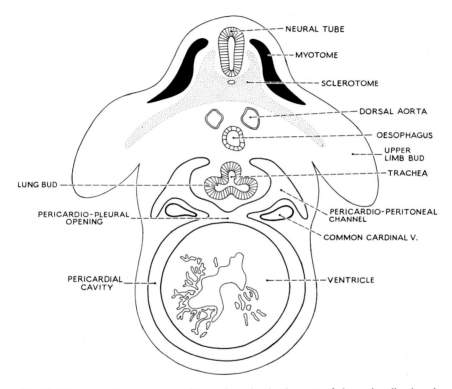

Fig. 52. Diagrammatic transverse section to show the development of the pericardio-pleural membranes by invagination of the lateral walls of the pericardio-pleural openings by the common cardinal veins.

wall and develops into the visceral pleura covering over the lung. Since the septum transversum is first found cephalic to the heart in the cervical region of the embryo, it receives a nerve supply from branches of the 3rd, 4th and 5th cervical nerves, which together constitute the phrenic nerve; the adult diaphragm is therefore innervated by the phrenic nerve, which consequently has a long course in the adult to reach its destination. The phrenic nerves utilize the pericardio-pleural membranes to reach the developing diaphragm and therefore lie on the adult fibrous pericardium (Figs 53, 55).

The pericardio-peritoneal canal does not develop into the whole of the pleural cavity; a secondary extension of it in a ventral direction lateral to the developing pericardial cavity forms the costo-mediastinal recess (Fig. 55), while an excavation of the lateral body wall produces the costo-diaphragmatic recess of pleura (Fig. 56). This excavation contributes tissue to the peripheral part of the diaphragm; since this is derived from the thoracic body wall it is therefore supplied by sensory fibres from the

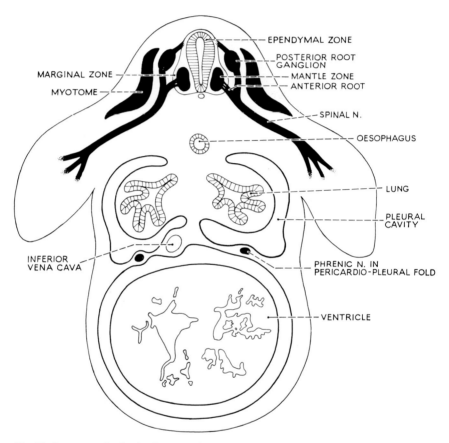

Fig. 53. Later stage in the development of the pericardio-pleural membranes. The pericardial cavity is now shut off from the pleural cavities.

intercostal nerves. The origin of the diaphragm is summarized in Fig. 54, which shows the contributions to this structure; the septum transversum, the pleuro-peritoneal membranes, the peripheral contributions from the body wall and the mesentery of the oesophagus all play a part.

Wells (1954) has described the development of the diaphragm and pleural sacs in great detail and gives an account of the formation of diaphragmatic hernias.

CLINICAL RELATIONSHIPS

Diaphragmatic hernia

A lack of closure of the left pleuro-peritoneal opening produced by a defect in formation of the left pleuro-peritoneal membrane results in one type of diaphragmatic hernia in 0·05% births. The defect is usually on the left side

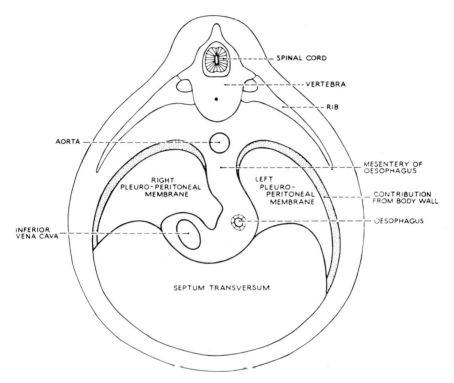

Fig. 54. Diagrammatic representation of a transverse section through an embryo to show the structures participating in the development of the diaphragm.

(85-90% cases) and is posteriorly situated, as can be seen from Fig. 54; it is sometimes termed the Foramen of Bochdalek, and allows the herniation of the stomach upwards into the thoracic cavity, when large enough. The defect can vary from a hole only 1 cm in diameter to complete absence of almost half of the diaphragm. Bilateral defects are most uncommon (1 in 60 cases). Other sites of diaphragmatic hernia are between the sternal and costal attachments of the diaphragm (Foramen of Morgagni, which occurs in 0·003% births) usually on the right side, and through the dome almost anywhere, but most commonly on the left side at the junction of the muscular and tendinous portions—i.e. at the junction between the part of the

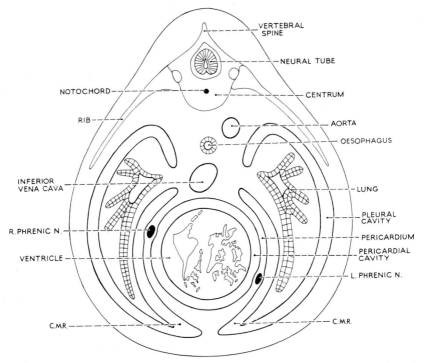

Fig. 55. A transverse section through the embryonic thorax at a stage later than that shown in Fig. 53 when the costo-mediastinal recesses (C.M.R.) have developed by excavation between the pericardium and body wall.

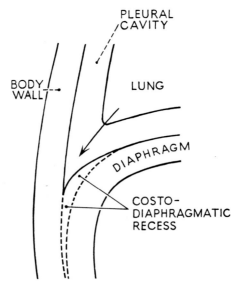

Fig. 56. A diagram illustrating the extension of the pleural cavity into the body wall to form the costo-diaphragmatic recess, so producing the periphery of the diaphragm.

diaphragm developed from septum transversum and other parts of the diaphragm. The commonest congenital diaphragmatic hernia, however, is an oesophageal hiatus hernia (0·05-0·08% births) usually of the "sliding" type, in which the cardiac region of the stomach prolapses through an enlarged oesophageal opening into the thorax. This is to be distinguished from the para-oesophageal hernia which is a true hernia on the right side of the oesophagus into the mediastinum (p. 95).

In the newborn a diaphragmatic hernia, particularly through the Foramen of Bochdalek, is recognizable by dyspnoea, cyanosis and the presence of gas filled loops of intestine in the thorax on X-ray. In the adult, depending on the size of the defect, the hernia may be asymptomatic or cause predominantly gastrointestinal symptoms. Primary surgical repair of the defect is necessary, with the aid of prosthetic materials in large defects.

The rarest type of diaphragmatic defect is in the central tendon, caused by abnormal development of the septum transversum. Only some dozen cases have been recorded and in all of them the anomaly leads to communication between the peritoneal and pericardial cavities.

The diaphragmatic pleura and the peritoneum under the diaphragm are innervated in a similar fashion to the diaphragm itself. Thus the pleura on the central part of the diaphragm, and the peritoneum under it, are supplied by the phrenic nerve and their irritation causes referred pain over the shoulder (C 3, 4 and 5 dermatomes). Irritation of the pleura or peritoneum related to the periphery of the diaphragm causes pain in the parts of the thoracic or abdominal wall supplied by the corresponding intercostal nerves.

Reference

Wells, L. J. (1954). Development of the human diaphragm and pleural sacs. *Contr. Embryol.* **35,** 107-134.

12

The Development of the Mouth and Nasal Cavities

Development of face

The appearance of the primitive stomodaeum formed by flexion of the head end of the embryo is shown in Fig. 57. It is bounded by the overhanging fore-brain, caudally by the bulging pericardial cavity and on each side by the mandibular and maxillary processes. Both of these processes develop from the first pharyngeal (mandibular) arch. In the depths of the stomodaeum lies the bucco-pharyngeal membrane. The maxillary process approximates to its fellow across the midline and there meets another process called the *frontonasal process,* a median bulge forming on the ventral aspect of the fore-brain. Meanwhile, however, the mandibular process rapidly contacts its fellow across the midline. Just above the maxillary process on each side, there are thickenings of the somatic endoderm overlying the brain, called the *nasal placodes.* These placodes sink into the lower end of the frontonasal process to form the *olfactory pits,* which thereby became bounded on each side by local elevations of the frontonasal process termed the medial and lateral nasal folds (Fig. 58). The lateral nasal fold forms the ala of the nose, whereas the medial nasal fold together with the remainder of the frontonasal process forms the dorsum and apex of the nose. As shown in Fig. 59, the maxillary process grows medially across the lower aspect of the olfactory pit, fuses first with the lateral nasal fold and then with the medial nasal fold. The two maxillary processes approximate to each other and first their epithelia and then the mesoderm of the processes fuse together to form the tissue of the upper lip. Since they are separated deeply by the mesoderm of the fronto-nasal process, this forms the deep tissue of the median part of the lip (the philtrum and adjoining tissue; see Fig. 60). In other words, the maxillary processes fuse together across the midline superficial to the lower aspect of the frontonasal process (see Warbrick, 1960). The mesoderm of the maxillary process must first fuse with the lateral aspect of the mesoderm of the frontonasal process, before the superficial tissue and epithelium of the maxillary processes override the lower end of the frontonasal process to form the upper lip.

Development of palate and nasal septum

While this is happening, each maxillary process also forms a horizontally directed shelf called the palatal process of the maxillary process, which grows across the cavity of the stomodaeum (Figs 61, 62), so dividing it into two

116

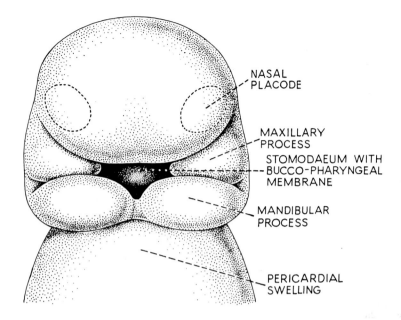

Fig. 57. The appearance of the stomodaeum of an early embryo from the ventral aspect showing the structures which bound this cavity.

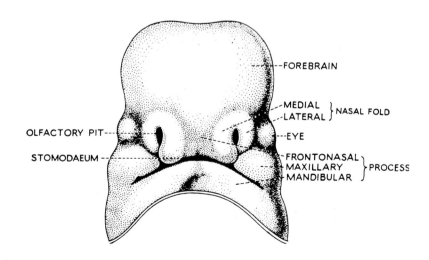

Fig. 58. Ventral aspect of the head of an embryo showing the olfactory pits and nasal folds.

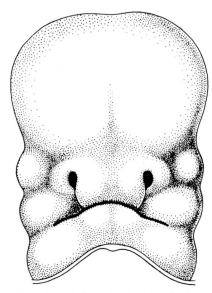

Fig. 59. Ventral aspect of the embryonic head showing growth of the maxillary processes in a medial direction across the lower aspect of the olfactory pits to contact and fuse with the medial nasal folds.

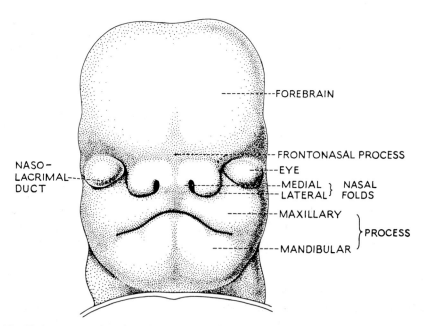

Fig. 60. Appearance of the face of an embryo after the maxillary processes have fused with the lower part of the frontonasal process to form the upper lip. The frontonasal process develops into the deep tissue of the median part of the lip, shown in stipple.

parts, an upper nasal cavity and a lower mouth cavity and fuses with its fellow (Fig. 63) to form a large portion of the palate; in the early stages of their growth the palatal processes are separated by the tongue (Fig. 61), but later fuse together above it. Intramembranous ossification in these processes forms the palatine processes of the maxilla in the adult. Inside the

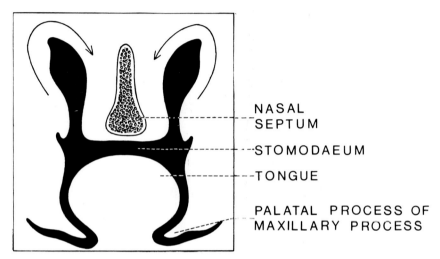

NASAL
SEPTUM

STOMODAEUM

TONGUE

PALATAL PROCESS OF
MAXILLARY PROCESS

Fig. 61. Coronal section through the developing stomodaeum to show the palatal processes growing medially towards each other, but separated by the tongue. The arrows show the direction of growth of mesoderm from the maxillary processes, constituting the tecto-septal extension which contributes to the nasal septum.

mandibular process is the cartilage of the first pharyngeal arch, called *Meckel's cartilage,* around which mesoderm condenses; this mesoderm undergoes intramembranous ossification to form the mandible, but Meckel's cartilage itself later atrophies and disappears except for certain structures (p. 213) and takes no part in the formation of the mandible. A cartilage in the maxillary process, the pterygoquadrate (palatoquadrate) bar, similarly provides the basis around which the maxilla ossifies intramembranously. Mesoderm covered with ectoderm grows dorsally from the deep aspect of the frontonasal process in the median plane of the stomodaeum as the rudiment of the nasal septum, which contacts the fused palatal processes of the maxillary processes inferiorly where the latter themselves meet and fuse. Some of the tissue which forms the septum may be derived from the maxillary process and migrates up the lateral wall of the stomodaeum as the *tectoseptal extension* to meet its fellow in the midline of the roof (see Fig. 61). The frontonasal process now sends a growth backwards in the same plane as the palatal processes of the maxillary processes. This is called the *primitive palate* and it differentiates into a part of the palate often called the premaxilla. Wood, Wragg and Stuteville (1967) have claimed that there is no independent centre of ossification for this part of the palate and that the premaxilla does not exist as an independent bone in man. It fuses on each side with the palatal processes of the maxillary processes, which form the largest part of the palate. The palate therefore consists of three elements. The most posterior part of the palatal processes does not ossify and so develops into the soft palate and uvula (Fig. 64). There is some ossification posterior to the palatine processes of the maxilla to form the palatine bones.

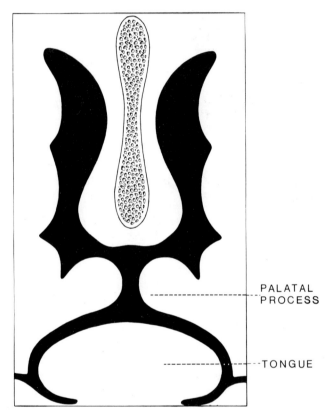

PALATAL
PROCESS

TONGUE

Fig. 62. Coronal section of the developing stomodaeum to show the approximation of the palatal processes above the tongue.

Each of the three processes which participate in the formation of the face has its own nerve supply and therefore in the adult there are definite territories of sensory innervation from the three divisions of the trigeminal nerve. This correlation is shown in Fig. 112 (p. 214). The serial histological changes in the development of the face and palate from 33 days to birth have been illustrated by Kraus, Kitamura and Latham (1966).

Streeter (1948) has claimed that it is better to consider the facial processes as swellings or ridges that correspond to centres of growth in the underlying mesoderm; although in the formation of the palate edge-to-edge fusion of the palatal processes must first occur, ectoderm is not absorbed between continuous surfaces of the facial processes but the furrows become shallower and smooth out as the increase in mass of tissue produces new levels. The

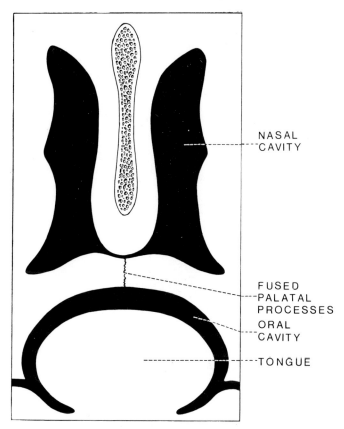

Fig. 63. Fused palatal processes at a later stage of development of the stomodaeum, separating the nasal and oral cavities. The lower end of the nasal septum has almost contacted and fused with the fused palatal processes.

term "process" should therefore be abandoned and the expression "growth centre" or ridge, or septum, for example, used instead (Harrison, 1957). Jacobs (1964) has shown that the competence of the embryological mechanism of palate closure is related to the developmentally normal relative increase of sulphated mucopolysaccharides, which act as a factor maintaining maximum visco-elasticity and minimal swelling of palatal processes.

Angelici and Pourtois (1968) in observing the fusion of palatal processes in rodents, found first a stickiness and then fusion of ectodermal epithelial cells over the processes to form a partition; this ectodermal partition then ruptured, allowing underlying mesenchyme from either side to contact its fellow and finally there was degeneration of the epithelial remains of the seam, marking the completion of fusion. The rupture of the partition is effected by enzymes, produced by lysosomes.

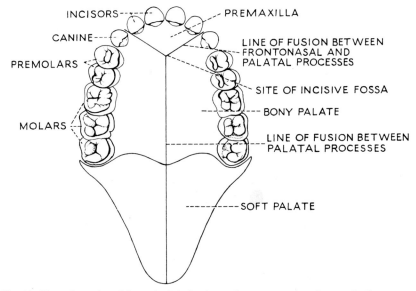

Fig. 64. The palate, viewed from the inferior (ventral) aspect, to show its constitution.

CLINICAL RELATIONSHIPS

Cleft palate

Defective fusion between the primitive palate and the palatal processes of the maxillary processes results in either a unilateral or bilateral *cleft palate*. If both palatal processes fail to reach the midline and fuse together, the lower free border of the nasal septum is visible in the resultant defect when viewed from the oral aspect. Such a median defect may involve only the soft palate or uvula, so producing a bifid uvula. It is known that one palatal process may succeed in reaching the midline to fuse with the nasal septum, whereas the other does not. In this case the oral cavity only communicates with one nasal cavity through the palatal cleft. Should the primitive palate only fail to fuse with one palatal process, a smaller degree of unilateral cleft palate results: failure of such fusion on both sides produces a bilateral cleft palate, the premaxilla being isolated in the anterior aspect of the roof of the mouth.

Such a defect is rare, however, since defective fusion of the primitive palate with the palatal processes is usually associated with failure of fusion between the palatal processes themselves.

Infants with cleft palate usually present with a severe nursing problem, since milk taken into the mouth often passes through the palatal defect into the nasal cavity, and may then be aspirated into the lungs. The defect also makes it extremely difficult for the babe to suck efficiently. Experienced nursing is necessary until the babe is sufficiently mature for a surgical repair of the palate defect.

Hare-lip

Cleft palate is often associated with hare-lip (cleft lip). This may also be either unilateral or bilateral (Fig. 65) when the maxillary process of one side or both sides fails to fuse with the lateral aspect of the frontonasal process. In bilateral hare-lip the region of the upper lip, formed from the frontonasal process, is visible in between the two lip defects. In median hare-lip the maxillary processes have failed to progress further, superficial to the lower aspect of the frontonasal process, to meet and fuse together in the midline. The maxillary process fuses with the side of the frontonasal process along a line in the adult drawn from the medial canthus of the eye to the ala of the nose. Failure of fusion here forms an *oblique facial cleft* (Fig. 65); in the depths of this an open nasolacrimal duct is exposed, since this normally develops by a sinking in of the groove at the site of fusion of maxillary and frontonasal processes. *Macrostomia* or *microstomia* may also occur as anomalies caused by relative lack of fusion or too much fusion between the maxillary and mandibular processes. Defective fusion or malfusion of the mandibular processes is very rare, and produces a median cleft in the chin; this may be associated with a midline defect in the underlying mandible.

The philtrum is the midline vertical groove in the upper lip and is said to be produced by the heaping up of maxillary process mesoderm at its lateral margins at the site of fusion between these processes and the frontonasal process. Mesoderm of the second pharyngeal arch follows the growth of maxillary and mandibular processes and differentiates into the musculature of facial expression. It follows, therefore, that if the maxillary processes are unable to fuse together over the lower aspect of the frontonasal process, the region of the upper lip between the defects of a bilateral hare-lip will be devoid of muscle tissue, and such is the case.

In certain experimental animals the administration of glucocorticoids such as cortisone to pregnant animals induces cleft palate in the offspring. Various inbred strains of mice show differing degrees of susceptibility to clefting in this way. This is probably related to the degree of affinity of glucocorticoid binding proteins in the cytoplasm of mesenchyme cells in the various facial processes. Cortisone is also known to inhibit the growth of embryonic and adult fibroblasts in both rats and mice, and the inhibition of

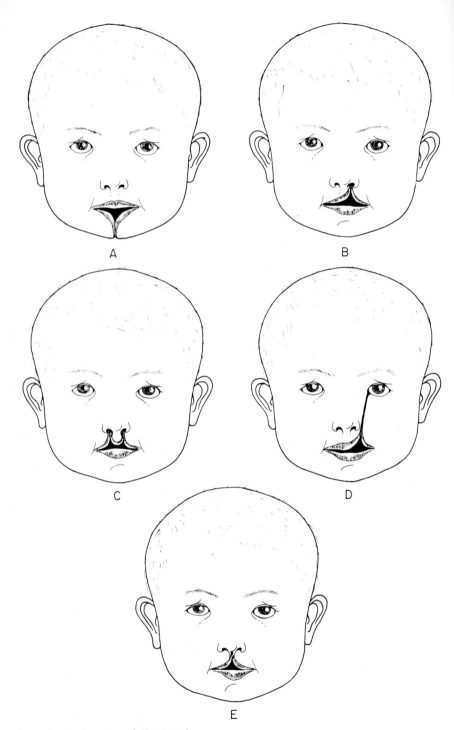

Fig. 65. (For legend see facing page.)

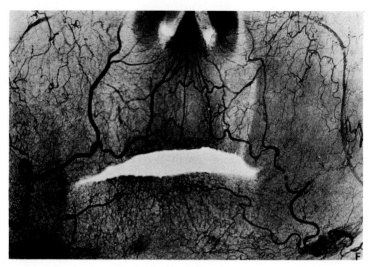

Fig. 65. Abnormalities in the development of the face. A. A median cleft of the lower lip and chin. B. A unilateral complete cleft lip. C. A bilateral complete cleft lip. D. An oblique facial cleft. E. A median cleft of the upper lip. F. An arteriograph showing the arteries supplying the lips. The pattern of distribution of arteries to the upper lip clearly reflects its developmental origin; kindly supplied by Mr D. C. Herbert, F.R.C.S.

proliferation of mesenchyme cells in the developing palate may well be a factor in the production of cleft palate. For these reasons the administration of corticosteroids such as hydrocortisone to a pregnant woman is to be condemned.

There are definite differences in the incidence of cleft palate in racial groups. In Baltimore, U.S.A., the rate for negro children with clefts was 0·55 per 1000 live births, but 1·06 per 1000 in Caucasians (Warkany, 1971). In Northumberland and Durham it was 1·4, in Denmark 1·5, in Sweden 1·75, in Birmingham 1·76, in Japan 2·7 and among Montana Indians 3·6 per 1000. These differences are not a purely racial characteristic, however, since the populations compared differ in environmental conditions. Left-sided cleft palate is more common than a right sided or bilateral clefts. Unilateral hare-lip occurs once in 2500 births and is bilateral in 15% cases. Hare-lip is three times as common in boys, but cleft palate is commoner in girls.

Surgical operations for repair of cleft palate are undertaken between six and eighteen months of age. Hare-lip is usually operated upon earlier, often as early as two to three months. In repair of hare-lip it is important to restore continuity of the orbicularis oris muscle. In the operation for repair of cleft palate, flaps of mucoperiosteum are elevated from the hard palate and stitched together over the defect. The hamulus of the medial pterygoid plate may have to be broken on each side in order to relax the tensor palati muscles.

In plastic surgery of the face great care must be taken to ensure that flaps of skin mobilized to repair defects have an adequate arterial supply. Formerly such operations were based on blood supply from the facial artery, but it is now known that the cheek, and particularly the region of the nasolabial sulcus, depends in large part on blood supply from the transverse facial branch of the superficial temporal artery (Herbert and Harrison, 1975), which may be regarded as an artery supplying the facial tissue derived from the maxillary process. The distribution of arteries to the upper lip (Fig. 65F) shows a pattern which reflects its developmental origin.

Hare-lip and cleft palate occasionally present as an inherited disorder showing male sex-linkage. When cleft palate occurs alone, the disorder may be due to a dominant gene of low penetrance. The defect may be accompanied by some other anomaly, such as Down's Syndrome, and often follows rubella infection of the mother during the first trimester of pregnancy.

The Pierre Robin syndrome is an association of cleft palate, the cleft usually being posteriorly situated, with under-development of the mandible (retrognathos) and consequent backward displacement of the tongue. The danger of this disorder is that the infant might die from respiratory obstruction because the tongue may fill the pharynx. Operative intervention to stitch the tongue more anteriorly in the mouth is therefore essential.

References

Angelici, D. and Pourtois, M. (1968). The role of acid phosphatase in the fusion of the secondary palate. *J. Embryol. exp. Morph.* **20**, 15-23.

Harrison, R. J. (1957). Nature and nurture in jaw development. *Dental Practitioner* **7**, 350-360.

Herbert, D. C. and Harrison, R. G. (1975). Nasolabial subcutaneous pedicle flaps. *Br. J. Plastic Surg.* **28**, 85-89.

Jacobs, R. M. (1964). S^{35}—liquid—scintillation count analysis of morphogenesis and teratogenesis of the palate in mouse embryos. *Anat. Rec.* **150**, 271-278.

Kraus, B. S., Kitamura, H. and Latham, R. A. (1966). "Atlas of Developmental Anatomy of Face" Harper and Row, London.

Streeter, G. L. (1948). Developmental horizons in human embryos: age groups XV, XVI, XVII and XVIII, being the third issue of a survey of the Carnegie collection. *Contr. Embryol.* **32**, 133-203.

Warbrick, J. G. (1960). The early development of the nasal cavity and upper lip in the human embryo. *J. Anat.* **94**, 351-362.

Warkany, J. (1971). "Congenital Malformations" Year Book Medical Publishers, Chicago.

Wood, N. K., Wragg, L. E. and Stuteville, O. H. (1967). The premaxilla: embryological evidence that it does not exist in man. *Anat. Rev.* **158**, 485-489.

13

The Heart

The parts of the intraembryonic coelom immediately caudal to the pericardial cavity formed in the protocardiac area join together ventral to the foregut and themselves contribute to the formation of the pericardial activity, by communicating with each other as well as with the original unpaired pericardial cavity (Fig. 66). The procedure whereby the pericardial cavity comes to lie on the ventral aspect of the foregut is assisted by flexion of the head end of the embryo. During this process, two endocardial heart primordia appear in a manner similar to the formation of the vascular system anywhere else in the body.

Blood vessels appear in the embryo in the splanchnopleuric extraembryonic mesoderm covering the yolk sac. Here equipotential cells called *angioblasts* congregate together to form islands of cells and eventually divergent differentiation (Weiss, 1953) in these islands results in the outer cells forming vascular endothelium and the inner ones free blood cells, the resultant structures being termed *angiocysts*. These then join up with one another to form longitudinal channels, the primitive blood vessels.

The heart tube

Exactly the same process occurs in the formation of the primitive *endocardial heart tubes*. Angiocysts develop in the space between the splanchnopleuric intraembryonic mesoderm and the endoderm of the yolk sac at the sides of the foregut. These differentiate from angioblasts which develop both from foregut endoderm and from splanchnopleuric intraembryonic mesoderm. The angiocysts undergo confluence in order to form a single endocardial heart tube on each side. The progressive lateral flexion of the embryonic plate, which ensures that the intraembryonic coeloms are approximated and fuse together to form the pericardial cavity, also enables the endocardial heart tubes to be brought together and fuse on the ventral aspect of the foregut (Fig. 66). This necessitates the pinching off of the foregut from the yolk sac in a transverse plane. Because the splanchnopleuric intraembryonic mesoderm in this region differentiates into the myocardium and epicardium of the heart, it is called the *myoepicardial (epimyocardial)* mantle; this contacts and fuses with its fellow around the endocardial heart tubes by a process which is very similar to that occurring in the gut, where the splanchnopleuric intraembryonic mesoderm approximates to form the mesenteries and the muscular and connective tissue around the gut. The myoepicardial splanchnopleuric intraembryonic mesoderm also forms a

127

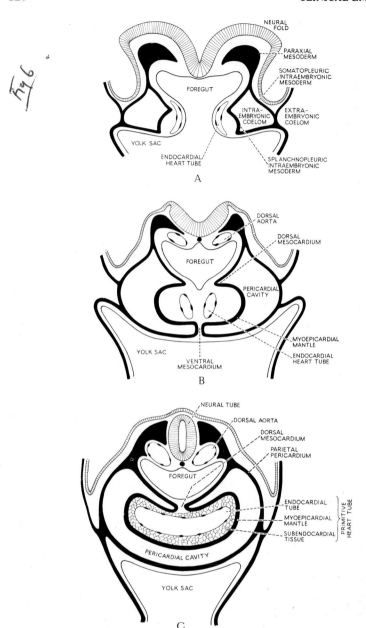

Fig. 66. The development of the heart from two endocardial heart tubes which appear in between the splanchnopleuric intraembryonic mesoderm and the endoderm of the yolk sac, is shown in A. These fuse together ventral to the foregut as shown in B, accompanied by approximation of the splanchnopleuric intraembryonic mesoderm to form the myoepicardial mantle and the dorsal and ventral mesocardia. Eventually the single primitive heart tube, shown in C, is suspended by the dorsal mesocardium, from the floor of the foregut in the pericardial cavity formed by fusion of the two intraembryonic coeloms.

mesentery, called the dorsal mesocardium, which attaches the primitive heart to the ventral aspect of the foregut. Once the endocardial heart tubes have fused together to form a single endocardial heart tube, which has become surrounded by a myoepicardial mantle, the whole can be considered as a single tube, the primitive heart tube, and the changes now to be described occur in both the endocardial and myoepicardial components.

The primitive heart tube is suspended by the dorsal mesocardium ventral to the foregut in the pericardial cavity (Fig. 67). The somatopleuric intra-embryonic mesoderm forms the parietal pericardium, while the splanchno-pleuric intraembryonic mesoderm develops into the visceral pericardium covering over the heart. In between the endocardial heart tube and the myoepicardial mantle is a loose reticulum of connective tissue called *sub-endocardial tissue*. Since the endocardium of the heart is formed in exactly the same way as the endothelium of blood vessels elsewhere in the embryo it is continuous caudally with veins entering the heart and cephalically with the arteries leaving it. The points where the primitive heart tube leaves the pericardial cavity at its cephalic and caudal aspects are relatively fixed, and when further growth of the heart takes place, it can only bend or buckle because of its fixation at the extremities of the pericardial cavity. While the bending of the heart tube is proceeding in a ventral direction, differential dilatation of the heart tube also occurs. The result of this process is the formation of several separate chambers called in order in a cephalo-caudal direction the *bulbus cordis, ventricle, atrium* and *sinus venosus* (Fig. 67). The ventricular end of the bulbus cordis is sometimes termed the conus and the cephalic end the truncus arteriosus. The sinus venosus consists mainly of two parts which have not yet undergone fusion and are termed respectively the right and left horns of the sinus venosus.

The most pronounced loop, which is formed in a ventral direction and slightly to the right, occurs between the bulbus cordis and the ventricle; this is the bulbo-ventricular loop. The atrium is carried on to the dorsal aspect of the ventricle and to the cephalic aspect of the pericardial cavity. A spiral septum forms inside the bulbus cordis and divides it into two parts, a primitive aorta and pulmonary artery, while the caudal aspect of the bulbus cordis becomes absorbed into the cavity of the ventricle, so enlarging the ventricular cavity which becomes divided by the *interventricular septum* into two ventricles. The common atrial cavity is divided into two atria by the formation of septa. The left horn of the sinus venosus grows very slowly and forms the coronary sinus, while the right horn takes predominance, due to the greater degree of development of systemic veins on the right side of the embryo and becomes absorbed into the right side of the primitive atrium; the systemic, umbilical and vitelline veins come to drain only into the right horn of the sinus venosus.

The changes that occur in these various chambers of the heart will be considered independently but it must be remembered that this is merely for

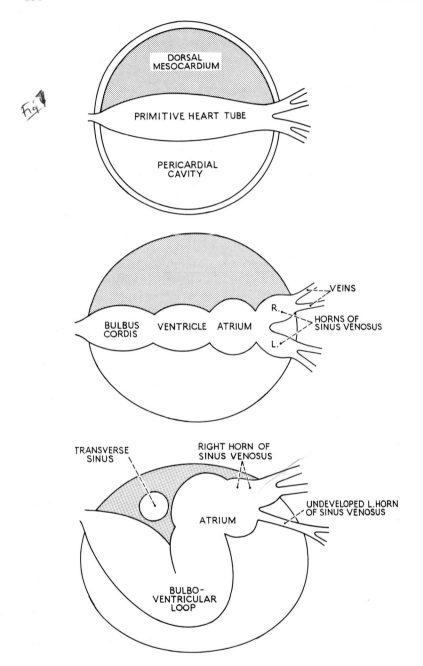

Fig. 67. Diagrammatic representation of the development of the primitive heart tube as seen from the left side.

convenience and that many of the developmental changes in the heart proceed simultaneously.

Development of the atria

The development of the common atrium can best be understood by examining it in coronal section (Fig. 68). The atrium leads inferiorly into a narrowed canal, the common *atrio-ventricular canal;* subendocardial tissue proliferates all around the opening of this canal, so that it becomes surrounded by a ridge of this tissue which has pushed up the endocardium to form the *atrio-ventricular cushions.* The right horn of the sinus venosus opens into the right side of the common atrium and the opening is bounded by two valves, *the right and left venous valves,* which fuse superiorly to form a septum called the *septum spurium*; this opening is called the sinu-atrial opening. The right venous valve grows by an increasing invagination of the right horn of the sinus venosus into the atrium but the left venous valve probably has its origin in a delamination of the *septum primum* (Odgers, 1935) which is concerned in the division of the common atrium into two atria; this septum grows downwards from the roof of the common atrial chamber towards the atrio-ventricular cushions and a foramen is formed between its lower free border and the atrio-ventricular cushions called the *foramen (ostium) primum.* Before it meets and fuses with the atrio-ventricular cushions, there is a local failure of growth of the septum primum in its upper part in order to form another foramen called the *foramen (ostium) secundum* (Odgers, 1935). The part of the atrio-ventricular cushions with which the septum primum fuses is actually in the middle of the common atrio-ventricular canal at a point where the dorsal and ventral atrio-ventricular cushions fuse together across it, so dividing it into two channels, the right and left atrio-ventricular canals. In other words, the septum primum meets and fuses with the fused atrio-ventricular cushions approximately in the median plane of the heart. When the foramen secundum has been formed, a second thicker and stronger septum, the *septum secundum,* grows on the right side of the septum primum, in the space between it and the septum spurium called the *interseptovalvular space* (Figs 68, 69). The fully developed inter-atrial foramen that results after formation of the septum secundum is called the *foramen ovale.* If the inter-atrial septum is examined from the right side it is seen that the lower free border of the septum secundum is concave downwards. Below this border the inter-atrial septum consists only of the septum primum. This embryological arrangement is reflected in the structure of the adult inter-atrial septum which has a limbus ovalis on its right surface below which is the fossa ovalis, the limbus representing the lower free border of the septum secundum. The foramen ovale is a channel by means of which the right and left atria are kept in communication throughout the whole of fetal life. Only after birth are the two septa apposed and the foramen closed.

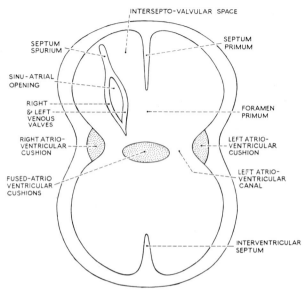

Fig. 68. A diagram of a coronal section through the heart viewed from the ventral aspect showing the development of the septum primum, sinu-atrial opening, atrio-ventricular cushions and interventricular septum.

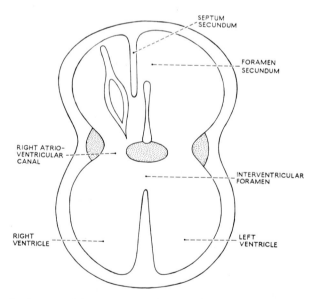

Fig. 69. The development of the septum secundum in the intersepto-valvular space on the right side of the septum primum which has grown towards, and fused with, the fused atrio-ventricular cushions separating the atrio-ventricular canals, and broken down in its upper aspect to form the foramen secundum.

Ventricular development

The first alteration in the common ventricular chamber is caused by the formation of a septum which grows upwards towards the atrio-ventricular cushions from the apex of the ventricle. This *interventricular septum* does not quite meet the atrio-ventricular cushions, so that for a while a foramen remains between them and the upper free border of the interventricular septum called the *interventricular foramen* (Fig. 70). At the same time, proliferation of subendocardial tissue in the bulbus cordis produces ridges

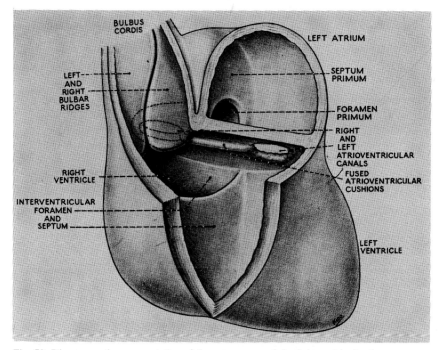

Fig. 70. Diagrammatic representation of the appearance of the interventricular foramen seen obliquely from the left ventral aspect following the removal of the left wall of the bulbus cordis and of the left atrium and part of the ventral wall of the left ventricle.

called the bulbar cushions or *bulbar ridges,* which are disposed right and left in the proximal part of the bulbus cordis, then anterior and posterior in the middle of this chamber and finally left and right in the topmost part of this chamber. This orientation is probably caused by the streamlining of blood flow from the two ventricles into the bulbus cordis. In fact, the bulbar ridges are probably produced as a result of moulding of subendocardial tissue in the bulbus cordis by the blood streams from the two ventricles, rather than by an actual proliferation of this tissue. The bulbar ridges fuse to form the aortico-pulmonary septum, which is the spiral septum dividing the bulbus cordis into ascending aorta and pulmonary artery; as a result the pulmonary artery twists around the ascending aorta in a spiral fashion in the adult heart. During this developmental change the axis of the whole heart rotates so that the right ventricle comes to lie ventral to the left ventricle. This rotation possibly occurs as a result of coincidental enlargement of the right lobe of the liver.

The bulbar ridges in the proximal part of the bulbus cordis are closely related to the atrio-ventricular cushions and all of them are in close relationship to the interventricular foramen. Proliferations from all of these structures close the interventricular foramen (Odgers, 1938); because they consist of subendocardial tissue, the part of the interventricular septum formed as a result of closure of the foramen is composed of fibrous tissue and constitutes the *pars membranacea septi* of the adult interventricular septum (Fig. 71). An important consequence of this process is that the anterior channel formed from the bulbus cordis, namely the pulmonary artery, is in communication with the right ventricle, whereas the posterior channel (the aorta) communicates with the left ventricle. Similarly, because the atrio-ventricular cushions fuse in the median plane of the heart, the two atrio-ventricular canals communicate with their corresponding ventricles.

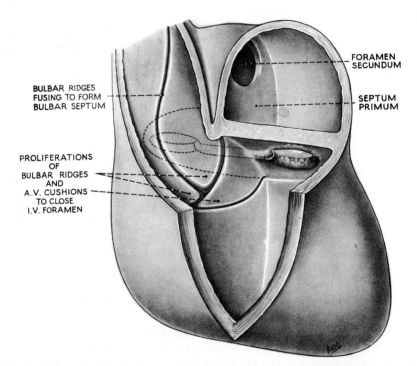

Fig. 71. Diagram showing the closure of the interventricular foramen by proliferations from the bulbar ridges and atrio-ventricular cushions to form the pars membranacea septi.

The various embryological tissues develop into clearly defined tissues in the adult heart. The endocardial heart tubes become the endocardium, while the myoepicardial mantle forms the muscular tissue and epicardium of the heart. Subendocardial tissue develops into fibrous tissue in the adult heart; the atrio-ventricular cushions, for example, form the valves in association with the left and right atrio-ventricular canals, the mitral and tricuspid valves. The ventricular extremities of the bulbar ridges develop into the aortic and pulmonary valves (Odgers, 1939). It has already been noted that the pars membranacea septi of the interventricular septum consists of fibrous tissue and is also formed from subendocardial tissue, all the proliferations from which produce noncontractile fibrous tissue composing the "heart skeleton", from which take origin and into which are inserted, directly or indirectly, all muscle fibres of the myocardium.

Later development of the right atrium

In later stages of development of the heart, the right horn of the sinus venosus becomes absorbed into the wall of the right atrium. Thus the adult right atrium develops from two structures. The most posterior part where the superior and inferior venae cavae enter (*the sinus venarum cavarum*) is derived from the right horn of the sinus venosus and is smooth on its internal aspect. The region of the adult right atrium derived from the right side of the primitive atrium is, however, lined by muscle bundles called musculi pectinati. These radiate from the *crista terminalis* (the remains of the septum spurium) which therefore marks the site of junction between the two parts of the right atrium; its position on the outside of the heart is indicated by the sulcus terminalis. The left venous valve fuses with the right side of the septum secundum and therefore contributes in part to the formation of the interatrial septum. The right venous valve becomes divided into two parts; the upper part forms the valve of the inferior vena cava, the lower part the valve of the coronary sinus. As a result of inclusion of the right horn of the sinus venosus in the right atrium, the superior and inferior venae cavae, which develop from systemic veins draining into the sinus, come to open directly into the adult right atrium. The left horn of the sinus venosus remains as the coronary sinus which lies in the atrio-ventricular groove, between left atrium and ventricle and opens into the right atrium.

CLINICAL RELATIONSHIPS

Both genetic and environmental factors are probably involved in the causation of congenital abnormalities of the heart. Since the Mongol child with its abnormality in chromosome distribution very often displays congenital heart disease, this is often taken as evidence that such anomalies can be inherited. One argument against inheritance of this disorder, however, is the fact that only one member of identical twins may be born with congenital heart disease, the other being perfectly normal. Rubella during the first three months of pregnancy is often a factor in the production of heart abnormalities in the offspring.

Situs inversus can affect the heart as well as other viscera. In addition, however, the heart alone may be situated with its apex pointing to the right instead of to the left (dextrocardia). Such a condition is, of course, compatible with a perfectly normal life. During development the heart "descends" relatively, due mainly to the straightening out of the curvature of the flexed embryo. Abnormal "descent" may be faulty in which case the heart comes to lie in the adult at a higher position than normal.

Since the development of the heart is quite complicated, anomalies of heart structure and orientation producing congenital heart disease, are common. Thus a persistent foramen ovale or patent interventricular foramen may occur and provide the means whereby abnormal admixture of arterial and venous blood in the heart takes place. Whenever a patent interventricular foramen occurs this is almost usually due (in 78% cases) to faulty development of the pars membranacea septi of the interventricular septum. Defects can also occur in the muscular part of the septum. Faulty division of the bulbus cordis may produce a narrowed pulmonary artery (pulmonary stenosis). This is often associated with an enlarged ascending aorta arising astride the upper part of the interventricular septum, since the interventricular foramen is patent, and a hypertrophy of the wall of the right ventricle (Fallot's tetralogy, which might more correctly be termed Fallot's tetrad since a tetralogy is a group of four Greek dramas). The resultant relative deoxygenation of arterial blood may be sufficiently severe as to cause cyanosis. Fallot's tetralogy is one of the most frequent congenital cardiac anomalies. The prognosis in this disease is good, although few patients live past the age of 40. By intracardiac surgery in suitable cases the pulmonary stenosis is treated by valvotomy and the ventricular septal defect repaired. Patent foramen ovale is just one form of atrial septal defect; maldevelopment of the septum primum or secundum may result in defects which persist in postnatal life and allow communication between the two atria. Atrial septal defects are among the most common congenital heart anomalies.

The foramen ovale may rarely close prematurely, so leading to increased work load and enlargement of the right ventricle. This prenatal closure of the foramen is often fatal and may be accompanied by severe oedema. Only some 20 cases are known, some due to lack of formation of the foramen secundum, others to excessive development of the septum secundum. Complete lack of development of the atrial septum or failure of large parts of the septum primum and septum secundum to develop, presenting as a large foramen primum, leads to cor triloculare biventricularis. A similar absence of the interventricular septum leads to cor triloculare biatriatum.

Septal defects can be treated by intracardiac surgery if sufficiently large as to lead to congestive cardiac failure and warrant operative intervention. The repair is effected by stitching together the edges of the defect or the insertion of a prosthetic patch in large defects.

Pulmonary stenosis may be so severe as to be represented as an atresia. The unequal division may similarly cause atresia or stenosis of the ascending aorta, or of the mitral or tricuspid orifices. The bulbar septum may be absent or partially defective, in which case there is either a common aortico-pulmonary trunk, or a communication between the aorta and pulmonary artery. The cardiac septa may be completely absent producing a heart which has one atrium and one ventricle (cor biloculare).

Defective development of the atrio-ventricular cushions is often associated with abnormal development of the mitral and tricuspid valves. Usually it is manifest as a result of defective fusion of the atrio-ventricular cushions with associated interatrial and interventricular septal defects. Often, however, the defective cushion development may be sufficiently severe as to result in a persistent common atrio-ventricular canal, which occurs in about 14% of cases of congenital cardiac disease. Excessive fusion of the atrio-ventricular cushions can result in either mitral or tricuspid atresia, in which the valve leaflets are fused. Such atresia leads to severe cyanosis and dyspnoea and is not amenable to treatment, because of an associated hypoplasia of the corresponding ventricle. The prognosis in valvular atresia is poor, infants often surviving only a few months at most after birth.

Aortic stenosis, which occurs in 2·3% of cases of major congenital heart lesions, may have a genetic basis when it is subaortic (i.e. below the level of the valve). When the stenosis is supravalvular it may be caused in certain families by doses of vitamin D which are well tolerated by the general population.

The overall incidence of congenital cardiac disease in babes born alive is 1%, but at least a third of these die before they are one year old. In the consideration of any form of congenital disease of the heart it is important to distinguish between anomalies (such as ventricular septal defects) caused by abnormal embryonic development during the critical period of cardiac differentiation in the fifth to seventh weeks, often caused by maternal rubella, and late defects occasioned by persistence of some part of the fetal heart or cardiovascular system which should have become non-functional and occluded after birth (e.g. persistent foramen ovale).

References

Odgers, P. N. B. (1935). The formation of the venous valves, the foramen secundum and the septum secundum in the human heart. *J. Anat.* **69**, 412-422.

Odgers, P. N. B. (1938). The development of the pars membranacea septi in the human heart. *J. Anat.* **72**, 247-259.

Odgers, P. N. B. (1939). The development of the atrio-ventricular valves in man. *J. Anat.* **73**, 643-657.

Weiss, P. (1953). Some introductory remarks on the cellular basis of differentiation. *J. Embryol. exp. Morph.* **1**, 181-211.

14

The Vascular System

DEVELOPMENT OF ARTERIAL SYSTEM

Since blood vessels develop in exactly the same way as the endocardial heart tubes, these tubes are continuous with veins at the caudal and arteries at the cephalic end of the primitive heart. Lower vertebrates such as the dogfish have a system of arteries supplying the branchial arches. This pattern is repeated in human development and, in the human embryo the *pharyngeal arch arteries* arise from the aortic sac, which is a continuation of the bulbus cordis, pass dorsally in the pharyngeal arches lateral to the pharynx and unite to form a dorsal aorta on each side. There is an artery (aortic arch) to each human embryonic pharyngeal arch; since there are six pharyngeal arches, there are six pharyngeal arch arteries (Fig. 72), but they do not all form at the same time. The first pharyngeal arch artery is the first to develop, since it lies in the cephalic end of the embryo, which is always precocious in its development. Almost as soon as it is differentiated it disappears and the second pharyngeal arch artery appears only to disappear very rapidly afterwards. This is followed by the appearance of the third and fourth pharyngeal arch arteries which persist but the fifth degenerates almost as soon as it forms. Finally the sixth pharyngeal arch artery develops and persists, so that the arch arteries to remain and form the adult arterial system are the third, fourth and sixth; they communicate the aortic sac, as it issues from the cephalic extremity of the bulbus cordis, with the dorsal aortae which are lying dorsolaterally on each side of the embryo. The manner in which the primitive arch arteries become modified to form the adult arterial system is illustrated in Fig. 73. The division of the bulbus cordis by the aortico-pulmonary septum also occurs in the aortic sac, which itself thereby becomes divided into ascending aorta and the stem of the pulmonary artery.

   The third arch artery on each side develops into the internal carotid artery; the continuation of the dorsal aorta into the head of the embryo forms the termination of this artery. The external carotid artery is a new vessel which develops by being drawn out from the aortic sac which also forms the common carotid artery in this way (Moffat, 1959). The left fourth arch artery persists and forms the arch of the aorta, and since the third and fourth arch arteries arise together from the aortic sac, the common carotid artery arises from the arch of the aorta. The sixth (Padget, 1954) cervical dorsolateral intersegmental artery (see p. 142) persists as a branch of the arch of the aorta, on the left side, to form the subclavian artery. On the right side, the parts of of the dorsal aorta between the third and fourth arch arteries and caudal to the fourth arch artery, completely disappear; the fourth arch artery on the right side therefore remains in direct communication with the sixth cervical dorsolateral intersegmental artery, the whole forming the right subclavian artery. The common origin of the right third and fourth arch arteries forms the brachiocephalic (innominate) artery, which in turn

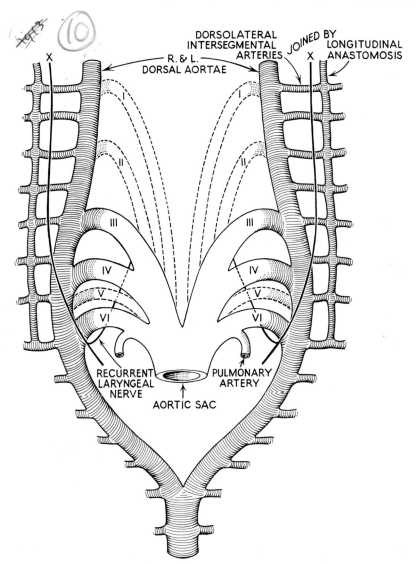

Fig. 72. Appearance of the pharyngeal arch arteries as seen from the ventral aspect. The vagus nerves (X) give origin to the recurrent laryngeal nerves which curve up behind the sixth pharyngeal arch arteries.

therefore arises from the arch of the aorta. From each sixth arch artery arises a branch which, with the proximal part of the artery on each side, develops into the pulmonary artery. But whereas on the right side, since the dorsal aorta disappears, the distal part of the sixth arch artery also disappears, on the left side it persists as a channel called the *ductus arteriosus* which connects the left pulmonary artery with the descending aorta. This important

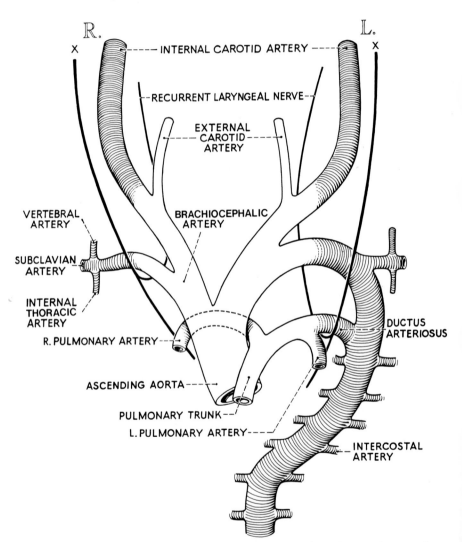

Fig. 73. The appearance of the arterial system of the embryo from the ventral aspect after modification of the pharyngeal arch arteries. Because the distal part of the right sixth arch artery atrophies, the right recurrent laryngeal nerve hooks around the right subclavian artery. On the left side, however, since this artery persists, the left recurrent laryngeal nerve hooks around the ductus arteriosus, and therefore around the adult ligamentum arteriosum.

channel communicates the pulmonary arterial circulation with the systemic arterial circulation throughout fetal life and only becomes closed soon after birth. It must not be confused with the ductus caroticus, which is the part of the dorsal aorta on each side in between the third and fourth pharyngeal arch arteries, undergoes closure, degenerates, and is of no functional significance. The division of the aortic sac occurs in the same plane as division of the fourth and sixth arch arteries, so that the aorta and its branches become separated from the pulmonary trunk and its two branches. The arterial system in man, therefore, predominates on the left side. This also occurs in other mammals but not uniformly so. Both dorsal aortae may persist in amphibia and reptiles, while in birds the arterial system predominates on the right side.

Branches of the aorta

From the aorta arise a series of vessels as shown in Fig. 74. They may be grouped into three classes:

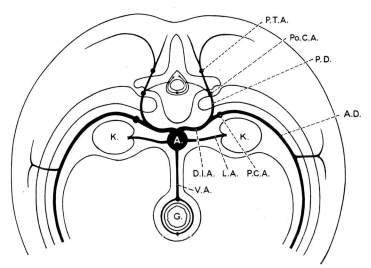

Fig. 74. Diagrammatic transverse section of an embryo through the region of the kidneys (K.), showing the branches of the aorta (A.). They are ventral arteries (V.A.) supplying the gut (G.), lateral segmental arteries (L.A.) to the intermediate mesoderm and dorsolateral intersegmental arteries (D.I.A.) to the body wall. The dorsolateral arteries have anterior (A.D.) and posterior (P.D.) divisions, precostal (P.C.A.), postcostal (Po.C.A.) and post-transverse (P.T.A.) anastomoses.

1. Ventral branches. These supply the primitive gut and are fundamentally the coeliac trunk, superior mesenteric artery and inferior mesenteric artery, and the regions of the gut which they supply have already been described (p. 53). These arteries are usually considered to be fundamentally paired arteries, arising in association with the paired intraembryonic coelom and when the two coeloms approximate (in much the same way as with the formation of the primitive heart tube), so do the blood vessels, fusing to form the median unpaired alimentary arteries. Also included in this group are the paired umbilical arteries; the fact that these two arteries remain paired is usually taken as evidence of the fact that the other ventral arteries were originally so. The two umbilical arteries are the main branches in the fetus of the aorta, the iliac arteries being merely branches of them. After birth, the umbilical arteries atrophy and, therefore, become themselves branches of the iliac arteries.

2. The lateral arteries. These supply the structures which develop in association with the intermediate mesoderm (intermediate cell mass), such as the adult kidneys, suprarenal glands and gonads; also to be included in embryonic life is the mesonephros. These arteries are fundamentally segmented, i.e. they are segmentally arranged one to each somite but as the kidneys and gonads become restricted to smaller areas large numbers of them disappear so that only a few branches remain to supply the adult structures.

3. The dorsolateral intersegmental arteries. These arise from the dorsolateral aspect of the aorta and almost immediately after their origin divide into two branches—a dorsal or posterior one, and a ventral or anterior one. The ventral branches course ventrally in the body wall as the intercostal and lumbar arteries. Various longitudinal (i.e. cephalo-caudal) anastomoses develop in relation to the ribs or costal elements of vertebrae. Each vertebra has a costal element. In the cervical region it forms the anterior root of the "transverse process", in the thoracic region a true rib, in a lumbar vertebra almost the whole transverse process and in the sacrum almost the whole of the lateral mass. There is one anastomosis in front of the head and neck of each rib which is therefore called precostal, one dorsal to the neck of the rib (post-costal), and one behind the transverse process termed post-transverse. The post-transverse anastomosis forms the deep cervical artery, while the precostal anastomosis develops into the thyro-cervical trunk and the highest intercostal artery. The post-costal anastomosis is very important since it develops particularly in the cervical region and forms the vertebral artery. It is continuous with the sixth cervical dorsolateral intersegmental artery inferiorly (Padget, 1954), which, as already noted, becomes the subclavian artery. The vertebral artery must come to lie in between the costal element and the true transverse process element of the so-called "transverse process" of the cervical vertebrae and in this position it occupies the foramina transversaria, which lie in between these two respective elements of the "transverse process". The proximal parts of the other dorsolateral cervical intersegmental arteries disappear completely and since none remain to connect with the aorta, the vertebral artery must take origin from the sixth cervical artery, namely the subclavian. This method of development of the vertebral arteries also explains the peculiar arrangement of the arterial supply of the spinal cord. The vertebral arteries in the foramen magnum give off anterior and posterior spinal arteries. No further major arterial branches are given off to the spinal cord in the cervical region but in the thoracic and lumbar regions the spinal arteries are contributed to by branches from the intercostal and lumbar arteries which remain intersegmental and whose post-costal anastomoses are homologous with the vertebral arteries.

Limb arteries

The arteries of limbs arise as a plexus of embryonic blood vessels within the limb buds. These become organized as an axis artery and then connect with the subclavian or iliac artery in the fore or hind limb bud, respectively. The axis artery only persists in part and is replaced by other vessels of the arterial limb plexus. Thus, in the forelimb, the axis artery perists as the axillary, brachial and anterior interosseous arteries; the radial and ulnar arteries arise late as new vessels from other limb plexus vessels (Fig. 75). The axis artery in the lower limb persists only as the inferior gluteal artery and its branch vascularising the sciatic nerve (*arteria comitans nervi ischiadici*), the popliteal and peroneal arteries (Fig. 76), since the femoral artery arises as a new vessel on the ventral aspect of the limb and largely takes over the arterial supply of the leg when it establishes communication with the iliac artery.

THE VENOUS SYSTEM

The venous system as it develops in the embryo can be divided into four parts:
    (a) Pulmonary venous system.
    (b) The systemic venous system, or cardinal system of veins.
    (c) The umbilical venous system.
    (d) The vitelline venous system which forms the portal system of veins.

One characteristic common to all mammalian embryos is the initial appearance of a bilaterally symmetrical pattern of primitive veins. This becomes transformed in later development presumably owing to genetic and haemodynamic factors (see Barnett, Harrison and Tomlinson, 1958).

Pulmonary venous system

The pulmonary veins could theoretically develop either as a diverticulum from the left atrium or by the formation of veins outside the left atrium with which they become secondarily connected; both processes in fact occur. The meshwork of veins formed in relation to the foregut and the component of this meshwork around the lung buds (Brown, 1913; Butler, 1952) forms four venous channels which link up to form two venous channels which then join and form a single pulmonary vein opening into an evagination of the left atrium (Auer, 1948; Los, 1958). The whole of this complicated system then becomes absorbed into the left atrium so that the four pulmonary veins then open into it independently. This governs the manner of reflexion of the pericardium around the pulmonary veins, as the oblique sinus of the pericardium. The common enclosure of the four pulmonary veins and the left atrium by pericardium is separated from a sleeve of pericardium surrounding the aorta and pulmonary artery by the transverse sinus of the pericardium which is brought about by a fenestration of the dorsal mesocardium. As

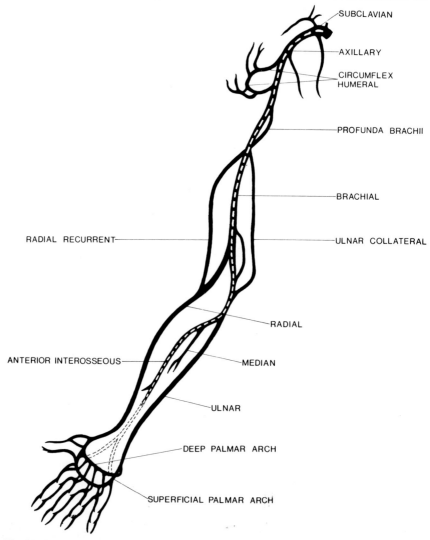

Fig. 75. The development of arteries of the forelimb. The position of the axis artery is shown in interrupted outline. It will be noted that the artery persists in great extent as the axillary, brachial and anterior interosseous arteries. Radial and ulnar arteries have arisen late as new vessels together with arteries of the hand.

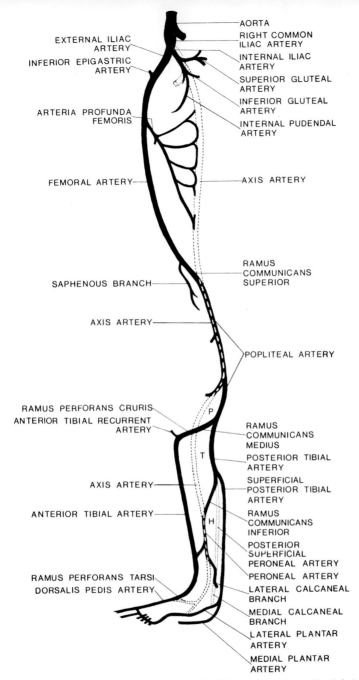

Fig. 76. Development of arteries of the hind limb. This persists only as the inferior gluteal artery, its branch which supplies the sciatic nerve, the popliteal and peroneal arteries. Large segments of the arteries have degenerated, and their situation is shown in dotted outline. The position of the popliteus muscle is shown at P., the tibialis posterior muscle at T. and the flexor hallucis longus muscle at H. It will be noted that even a secondary artery formed during the course of development (the posterior superficial peroneal artery) ultimately degenerates also. The femoral artery is the major new artery of the limb, and the dorsalis pedis artery arises to replace the ramus perforans tarsi.

shown in Fig. 67, this fenestration occurs in between the bulbus cordis and the atrium and therefore in the adult lies in between the pulmonary artery and the aorta in front and the left atrium behind. The transverse sinus is a much more important structure than the oblique sinus in the adult, since it acts as a "bursa" filled with pericardial fluid lying in between the aorta and the pulmonary artery anteriorly, which are pulsating asynchronously with the atrium lying behind the bursa.

Systemic venous system

In the development of the systemic venous system, there is a recapitulation of the venous system found in lower vertebrates. The first systemic veins to appear in human development are the anterior and posterior cardinal veins (Fig. 77). The posterior cardinal veins anastomose at the caudal end of the embryo. Each anterior cardinal vein joins with the ipsilateral posterior cardinal vein to form the common cardinal vein or *duct of Cuvier,* which opens into the corresponding horn of the sinus venosus. It has already been mentioned that the right horn of the sinus venosus takes predominance and that the left horn grows less rapidly to form the coronary sinus. It may be presumed that the venous system in consequence is predominant on the right side of the body and this is, in fact, what takes place, in complete contrast to the arterial system. First there is a cross-communication between the two anterior cardinal veins; since this anastomosis forms the left brachiocephalic vein it can be seen from Fig. 77 that something approximating to the arrangement of veins in the adult is produced. The right common cardinal and caudal part of the right anterior cardinal vein form the superior vena cava. Both anterior cardinal veins may, however, persist into adult life as paired superior venae cavae but normally the left common cardinal vein is very undeveloped and only remains as the oblique vein of the left atrium.

With increasingly complex vertebrate anatomy, a greater body size and more highly organized tissues, an increasingly complex venous system is evolved, since the more primitive types of venous pattern may be inadequate for their needs. When mesonephric kidneys develop, for example, and the vertebrate adopts a terrestrial environment, a system of veins must develop in order to drain its kidneys; this system of veins is called the subcardinal system and it is the next system to develop in the human embryo. Therefore, as soon as the mesonephroi develop in the human embryo, a pair of large *subcardinal veins* appears to drain these structures and they are in communication by means of an even larger inter-subcardinal anastomosis.

As a vertebrate becomes bigger and similarly as the human embryo grows larger, it must develop further systems of veins to drain its body wall which replace the posterior cardinal veins; these are the *thoracolumbar system* of veins (*supracardinal* or lateral sympathetic line system of veins, because they lie lateral to the sympathetic chain) and the *azygos system* of veins (or medial sympathetic line system of veins, see Reagan, 1927). An anastomosis

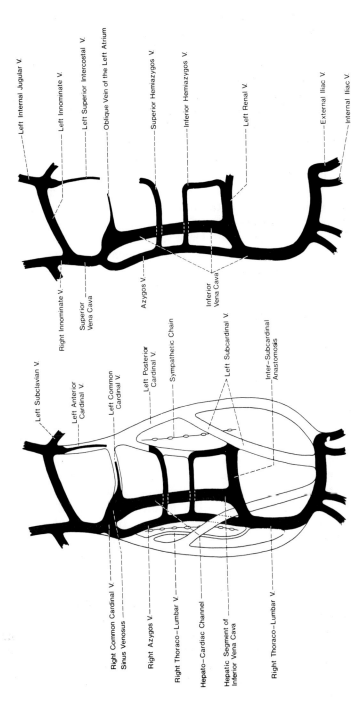

Left Internal Jugular V.
Left Innominate V.
Left Superior Intercostal V.
Oblique Vein of the Left Atrium
Superior Hemiazygos V.
Inferior Hemiazygos V.
Left Renal V.
External Iliac V
Internal Iliac V

Left Subclavian V.
Left Anterior Cardinal V.
Left Common Cardinal V.
Left Posterior Cardinal V.
Sympathetic Chain
Left Subcardinal V
Inter–Subcardinal Anastomosis

Right Innominate V.
Superior Vena Cava
Azygos V.
Inferior Vena Cava

Right Common Cardinal V.
Sinus Venosus
Right Azygos V.
Right Thoraco–Lumbar V.
Hepato–Cardiac Channel
Hepatic Segment of Inferior Vena Cava
Right Thoraco–Lumbar V.

Fig. 77. Diagram showing the modification of the embryonic systemic venous system to form the veins of the adult. The diagram on the left of the figure shows the complex of veins present in the early embryo: only those portions stippled persist to form the adult venous system shown on the right of the figure.

develops between the thoracolumbar vein and the right side of the inter-subcardinal anastomosis; an anastomosis also develops between this latter point and the right horn of the sinus venosus. From these arrangements, as can be seen from Fig. 77, the inferior vena cava is formed. The inferior vena cava therefore has a complicated origin: (a) the anastomosis between the inter-subcardinal vein and the right horn of the sinus venosus (the hepatic segment of the I.V.C.), (b) the right side of the inter-subcardinal anastomosis, (c) an anastomosis between the latter and the thoracolumbar vein, (d) the thoracolumbar vein itself and, finally, (e) the anastomosis between the posterior cardinal veins at the caudal end of the embryo, which forms the iliac veins. The inferior vena cava therefore develops on the right side of the embryo; also, a vein on the left side of the abdomen issuing from a viscus developed in association with intermediate mesoderm drains into the left renal vein which develops from the inter-subcardinal anastomosis, while a vein on the right side drains into the inferior vena cava. This is, in fact, what happens in the case of both the gonadal and suprarenal veins. The azygos system of veins develops into the system of the same name in the adult (see Butler, 1950) and the azygos vein, which is formed on the right side of the thorax, drains into the superior vena cava. For the same reasons, the lower end of the azygos vein in the adult is connected in the abdomen with the inferior vena cava, whereas the inferior hemiazygos vein connects directly or indirectly with the left renal vein.

Once this definitive venous system is established, all the other embryonic veins in the systemic system degenerate (Fig. 77).

Umbilical and vitelline systems

These two systems of veins develop in close association, the latter forming the portal system of veins. Figure 78 shows the liver from the ventral aspect; the left umbilical vein (the right having atrophied) approaches its lower border and towards the middle of the liver, two vitelline veins. These veins anastomose with each other at the lower surface of the liver (the sub-hepatic anastomosis) and also give off branches to the liver substance. At the superior surface of the liver, veins draining it pass into an infra-diaphragmatic anastomosis of veins and then into the inferior vena cava. These veins are called the *venae revehentes* and they form the hepatic veins, whereas the *venae advehentes* formed from the vitelline veins develop into the portal system of veins. The vitelline veins are first lying on each side of the duodenum. A cross-anastomosis develops between them in such a fashion that when the duodenum forms a loop which swings over to the right, the portal vein which develops from the vitelline veins adopts its adult relationship with the duodenum as shown in Fig. 79, since the lower anastomosis passes in front of the future horizontal part of the duodenum and the upper anastomosis between the two vitelline veins passes behind the superior part of the duodenum.

When the right horn of the sinus venosus starts to show predominance, a large channel called the *ductus venosus* appears in relation to the liver connecting the left umbilical vein with the right horn of the sinus venosus, by way of the inferior vena cava; its position is in or near the median sagittal plane (Dickson, 1957). This channel acts as a short circuit through the liver, enabling the blood returning from the placenta through the left umbilical

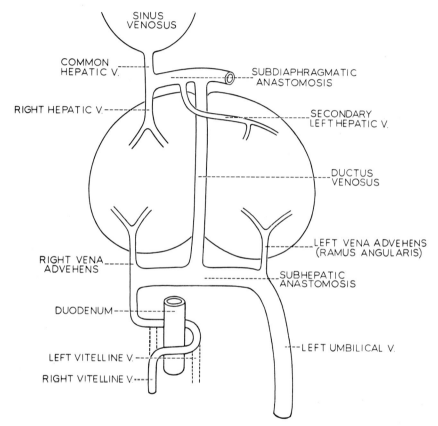

Fig. 78. Appearance of the venous circulation through the embryonic liver, seen from the ventral aspect, in early development.

vein to bypass the liver without losing any oxygen. As can be seen from Fig. 79, the portal vein opens into the right side of the liver. Throughout embryonic life the portal vein is not very important since digestion is not proceeding in the gut and therefore no food material needs to be transported from the gut to the liver. All food materials and oxygen reach the embryo through the left umbilical vein and consequently this blood vessel is very important indeed; after birth the left umbilical vein atrophies to form the ligamentum teres of the liver and the portal vein takes predominance. The right half of the sub-hepatic anastomosis becomes the *portal sinus* (Dickson, 1957), which connects the left umbilical with the portal vein in fetal life.

Haemopoiesis

Just as the first blood vessels are formed in the wall of the yolk sac, so also are blood cells formed in the same situation by the process of haemopoiesis. When the blood islands differentiate from the angioblasts, some of the cells

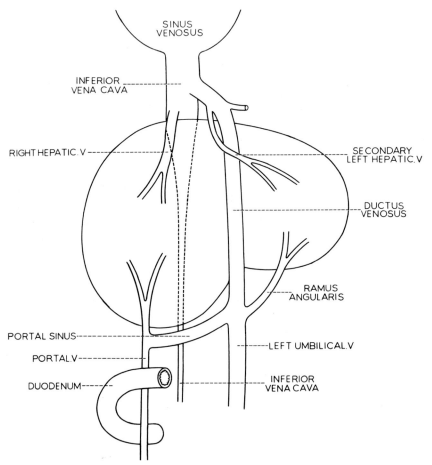

Fig. 79. The venous circulation through the embryonic liver in later development, seen from the ventral aspect.

at the periphery of the islands form the walls of the blood vessels but other central cells remain in the lumina of the blood vessels and produce blood cells. These cells are of a common type called haemocytoblasts and all of the fetal blood corpuscles are formed from these cells, including both erythrocytes and leucocytes. Transitional cell-types—erythroblasts in the formation of erythrocytes and promyelocytes and myelocytes in the production of leucocytes—are visible in the haemopoietic process. As blood vessels ramify throughout the connective tissue of the body, certain regions of the intra-embryonic connective tissue also become able to produce blood cells. For example, after blood corpuscles are formed in the yolk sac, the site of haemopoiesis changes to the liver, and then later on to the spleen, the mesonephros and finally to the bone marrow, the site of their production in post-natal life. Although lymphocytes can develop from haemocytoblasts, they are also produced in lymph nodes and in the thymus.

The lymphatic system

The development of lymphatics was investigated by Sabin (1912) who demonstrated that they are formed as diverticula from veins, and Huntington and McClure (1907) who claimed that they differentiate from clefts in the mesenchyme and only secondarily communicate with the venous system. Sabin showed that there are five lymphatic sacs formed as diverticula of the systemic veins. There are two jugular lymphatic sacs, diverticula of the internal jugular veins, two iliac lymphatic sacs formed as diverticula from the common iliac veins and a single median retroperitoneal unpaired lymph sac arising as a diverticulum from the inferior vena cava, which forms the cisterna chyli. These five lymphatic sacs then become interconnected by means of lymphatic channels. A cross-communication between the two anterior channels (which have formed in between the cisterna chyli and jugular lymph sacs) is responsible for the thoracic duct pursuing its characteristic adult course. This is almost certainly the method in which the major components of the lymphatic system develop; Huntington and McClure claimed that the more peripheral lymphatics are formed by clefts in the mesenchyme, which then connect with the main lymphatic channels. This view is not held by Yoffey and Courtice (1956) who claim that growth of embryonic lymphatic vessels is by endothelial sprouting in a centrifugal direction. The knowledge that the major lymphatics form as diverticula from veins also explains why the thoracic duct opens into the venous system anyway and the fact that in certain animals, for example the cat, lymphatics communicate at other sites with the venous system.

CLINICAL RELATIONSHIPS

Two aortae or a right-sided aorta may persist into adult life. The latter is, of course, associated with dextrocardia. In *transposition of the great arteries* the aorta arises from the right ventricle and the pulmonary artery from the left ventricle. This anomaly occurs once in 11,000 children below age 14 and is usually fatal, 85% affected children dying within six months after birth. In such cases the thoracic surgeon now performs a relocation operation, transferring the great vessels to connect with their normal ventricles; the great difficulty in this operation is the problem of transferring the coronary arteries with the aorta, but this has now been overcome. The operation must obviously be performed soon after birth, otherwise the left ventricle will diminish in size, having had to cope only with the smaller pulmonary circulation, and will be incapable of sustaining systemic arterial pressures.

If the ductus arteriosus remains patent, this provides a means whereby pulmonary and systemic arterial circulations mix. Patent ductus arteriosus is the most common congenital cardiac defect, and occurs in 1:5,500 children under the age of 14 years. The patent ductus can be completely divided surgically, taking care of the left recurrent laryngeal nerve. The process of fibrosis which normally eventually occludes the ductus before the end of the first year of life may extend to involve the aorta to produce a form of aortic stenosis termed *coarctation of the aorta*. In this common condition (in Sweden 0·62 per 1000 live births), the pulse in the femoral artery is either diminished or absent, and a large collateral circulation, involving mostly the intercostal arteries, is built up. Treatment is by surgical excision of the coarcted segment of the aorta and approximation of the cut ends.

The other large vessels which develop from aortic arches may similarly show abnormalities in pattern. This most frequently affects the subclavian and carotid arteries.

The pulmonary veins may open into the right atrium as a result of defective absorption of the right horn of the sinus venosus into the atrium. The left anterior and common cardinal veins may persist (as found in 1 out of 750 cadavers) to form a left superior vena cava. This may present together with a normal right superior vena cava. The hepatic segment of the inferior vena cava may be absent, and a double inferior vena cava is found in 2-3% persons. The venous anomalies are usually asymptomatic.

A bilateral inferior vena cava may similarly develop as a result of persistence of posterior cardinal veins on both sides. A single left sided inferior vena cava is also known, and is a natural accompaniment of dextrocardia. Because of the complicated origin of the inferior vena cava, many anomalies are known to occur in this vessel.

Blood disorders

There are many known congenital anomalies in the production of blood. Thus, there may be a defect in the formation of erythrocytes, which may be small and spherical—a disorder known as spherocytosis, or a defect in formation of haemoglobin, for example. The haemoglobin in the fetus differs from that in the adult, mainly owing to a difference in the globin of the haemoglobin molecule. In some Mediterranean people fetal haemoglobin may continue to be produced after birth, causing a type of haemolytic anaemia (Thalassaemia) which may be fatal. Haemolytic disease of the newborn (erythroblastosis fetalis) is a common disorder produced by incompatibility between parental Rh blood groups, the father being Rh positive and the mother Rh negative. Rh positive antigens are carried by fetal red cells across the placental barrier into the maternal circulation and stimulate the production of antibodies which pass back into the fetus and cause destruction of erythrocytes. The resultant haemolytic disease is manifest in several forms, such as icterus gravis neonatorum in which the haemolysed erythrocytes cause severe jaundice, or hydrops fetalis in which the child is stillborn and appears bloated with subcutaneous oedema. Elliptocytosis is another defect in the formation of erythrocytes which are shaped like rugby footballs. This condition is inherited as an autosomal dominant, and it may sometimes be associated with anaemia. The gene responsible for elliptocytosis may be linked to that controlling Rh blood groups, when it is harmless. The other form of this disorder causing anaemia, is not linked to the Rh gene.

Megakaryocytes also develop from haemocytoblasts and, if the red marrow is hypoplastic, these cells may be reduced or absent so that platelets are reduced in number (thrombocytopenia). Such congenital thrombocytopenia is usually found in children born of mothers with thrombocytopenic purpura. Red bone marrow hypoplasia which involves only the erythropoietic tissue but not granulocytopoietic tissue or megakaryocytes, can also be congenital, in which case the resulting disorder is congenital hypoplastic anaemia.

Lymphatic disorders

Congenital disorders in the development of the lymphatic system are not uncommon. A congenital hypoplasia of lymphatic vessels, usually in one or both legs, causes a pronounced oedema obvious at birth (Milroy's disease; hereditary lymphoedema). If the clefts in mesenchyme fail to unite with the major part of the lymphatic system formed by diverticula from the venous system, a cyst is formed—a condition termed cystic hygroma, and most common in the neck.

Anomalous vessels, whether they be arteries, veins or lymphatics are very common. Veins in particular show marked variation in their course, origin and termination. Such anomalies may be due to the persistence of vessels which should normally disappear, or the disappearance of vessels which should persist; in other words a lack of normal organization of the original network of vessels in an organ, limb or tissue.

References

Auer, J. (1948). The development of the human pulmonary vein and its major variations. *Anat. Rec.* **101**, 581-594.

Barnett, C. H., Harrison, R. J. and Tomlinson, J. D. W. (1958). Variations in the venous sysem of mammals. *Biol. Rev.* **33**, 442-487.

Brown, A. J. (1913). The development of the pulmonary vein in the domestic cat. *Anat. Rec.* **7**, 299-329.

Butler, H. (1950). The development of the azygos veins in the albino rat. *J. Anat.* **84**, 83-94.

Butler, H. (1952). Some derivatives of the foregut venous plexus of the albino rat with reference to man. *J. Anat.* **86,** 95-109.

Dickson, A. D. (1957). The development of the ductus venosus in man and the goat. *J. Anat.* **91,** 358-368.

Huntington, G. S. and McClure, C. F. W. (1907). The development of the main lymph channels of the cat in their relations to the venous system. *Am. J. Anat.* **6,** 36-41.

Los, J. A. (1958). "De embryonale ontwikkeling van de venae pulmonales en de Sinus Coronarius by de mens" Luctor´et Emergo, Leiden.

Moffat, D. B. (1959). Personal communication.

Padget, D. H. (1954). Designation of the embryonic intersegmental arteries in reference to the vertebral artery and subclavian stem. *Anat. Rec.* **119,** 349-356.

Reagan, F. P. (1927). The supposed homology of vena azygos and vena cava inferior considered in the light of new facts concerning their development. *Anat. Rec.* **35,** 129-148.

Sabin, F. R. (1912). On the origin of the abdominal lymphatics in mammals from the vena cava and the renal veins. *Anat. Rec.* **6,** 335-342.

Yoffey, J. M. and Courtice, F. C. (1956). "Lymphatics, Lymph and Lymphoid Tissue" Arnold, London.

15

The Fetal Circulation

The flow of oxygenated blood

The circulation of the blood around the fetal vascular system differs from that in the adult and therefore changes must occur in it at or immediately after birth. On returning from the placenta umbilical venous blood first approaches the liver. The arrangement of the vascular system of the liver is shown in Fig. 79. In fetal life the left umbilical vein approaches the centre of the liver and there divides into three main channels. The most important of these is a wide channel which is almost a direct continuation of the left umbilical vein and passes into the inferior vena cava. This channel is the ductus venosus and the opening into it is guarded by a sphincter; it short-circuits the liver and carries oxygenated blood directly from the placenta to the inferior vena cava and on into the heart. The second channel which is provided from the left umbilical vein is given off from its right side and links it with the portal vein; it is called the sinus intermedius or *portal sinus*. The direction of blood flow along this channel is from the left umbilical vein to the portal vein; the latter therefore vascularizes only the right third of the liver. The third branch of the left umbilical vein supplies the left third of the liver. The majority of the blood which returns from the placenta, therefore, bypasses the liver substance and flows directly into the inferior vena cava. After a very short course in the inferior vena cava, the oxygenated blood reaches the right atrium and here it impinges on the lower free border of the septum secundum. It is directed towards this lower concave border by the valve of the inferior vena cava and there divides into two streams. The larger of the two streams passes into the left atrium through the foramen ovale and through the left atrio-ventricular canal into the left ventricle to leave it by the ascending aorta. The first branches of the arch of the aorta being the brachiocephalic, common carotid and left subclavian arteries, the oxygenated blood which has come from the placenta is preferentially distributed to the coronary arteries and the head and neck and brain of the embryo, the regions which are developing most rapidly.

The flow of deoxygenated blood

The small portion of the stream which is diverted into the right atrium at the lower free border of the septum secundum joins the stream of deoxygenated blood passing down the superior vena cava into the right atrium. This stream courses into the right ventricle and then leaves it through the pulmonary artery. The course of this flow of blood has been elucidated by Barclay,

155

Franklin and Pritchard (1944), who investigated the fetal circulation of the lamb and followed the direction of blood flow by means of cineradiography. Because they found that the flow passing into the right atrium along the inferior vena cava is divided on the lower free border of the septum secundum, they termed this latter septum the crista dividens. The direction of the flow of blood passing down the superior vena cava into the right ventricle is governed by a tubercle which exists in between the orifices of the superior and inferior venae cavae which was first described by Lower (1669) and has been known since as the tubercle of Lower. Since it lies in between the superior and inferior venae cavae, Barclay, Franklin and Pritchard (1944) christened it the *crista interveniens*.

The deoxygenated blood issuing from the right ventricle through the pulmonary artery does not pass to any great extent into the lungs; they do not need a very great blood supply, since they are not functioning during fetal life. The main flow of blood along the pulmonary artery passes into its left branch and then into a channel which is mainly a continuation of this branch in fetal life, namely the ductus arteriosus, which developed from the left sixth pharyngeal arch artery (Fig. 80). By flowing along this channel, which is as wide as the aorta itself in fetal life, the deoxygenated blood reaches the descending aorta and by then flowing along its two main branches, namely the umbilical arteries, it reaches the placenta to be reoxygenated. Deoxygenated blood is bypassed through the ductus arteriosus into the descending aorta just beyond the arch and therefore does not supply the head and neck.

Changes at birth

After birth, the baby obtains its nourishment through its mouth and its oxygen through its lungs and therefore its circulation must change accordingly in order to adjust itself to the new demands. The first major physiological event after birth is that the baby respires. Its lungs become inflated and consequently there is a great fall in intrathoracic pressure (to as low as —50 mm mercury), a decrease in pulmonary vascular resistance and the rate of blood flow through the arterial circulation of the lungs increases five to ten fold within a few minutes (Born, Dawes, Mott and Widdicombe, 1954). It must then return through the pulmonary veins and this leads to an increase of pressure inside the left atrium, as a result of which the septum primum is apposed to the septum secundum and, therefore, the foramen ovale is closed. It used to be thought that the ductus arteriosus closes first, so that blood is therefore diverted into the terminal ramifications of the arterial circulation in the lungs. But it has been found by Barclay *et al.* (1944) and Born *et al.* (1954) that the foramen ovale always closes first. Indeed, closure of the ductus is not complete for many hours, during which time there is a *reverse* flow of blood along it, from aorta to pulmonary artery.

The other major event after birth is that the umbilical arteries constrict and this is only later followed by constriction of the left umbilical vein. It has been claimed that the umbilical cord should not be clamped or tied immediately after birth, because blood will pass through the left umbilical vein from the placenta for a period of time without the babe itself losing any blood; the baby may receive an additional quantity of blood equal to

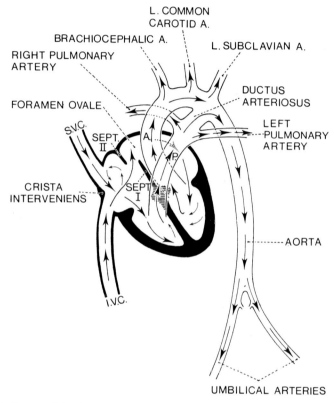

Fig. 80. A diagram of the circulation of the blood through the fetal heart. The arrows indicate the direction of flow of blood and their size gives an indication of the quantity of blood flowing. A. = Aorta. P. = Pulmonary trunk. Sept. I = Septum Primum. Sept. II = Septum Secundum.

0·8-4·7% of its body weight in this way (Gunther, 1957). Erythrocytes in the newborn child are later completely replaced by new blood corpuscles formed in the bone marrow, so the advantage to the fetus in obtaining an extra supply of blood from the placenta is that, when broken down, it provides a store of raw materials (for example, iron) which can be used for the formation of new blood. In normal babies, the systolic blood pressure falls significantly during the first 24 hours of life; delay in clamping the cord delays the fall, but does not affect its magnitude (Ashworth and Neligan, 1959).

The next thing to occur is "contraction" of the spleen immediately after the umbilical cord is tied (or, in certain other animals, ruptured). This may be in order to force red cells into the circulation to tide the fetus over the crucial moment when no further blood passes from the placenta to the fetus. When *contraction* of the spleen occurs after tying of the umbilical cord, this is only in such animals as the dog, which have smooth muscle in the capsule of the spleen. In the human being, however, there is very little smooth muscle and, therefore, any alteration in splenic volume must be produced by alteration in the distribution of blood within the spleen.

There is then a marked decrease in size of the liver, occasioned by the fact that there is no blood passing along the left umbilical vein to the left two-thirds of the liver and the portal vein has now to provide blood to the whole of the liver; since there is not an immediate pronounced increase in circulation of blood through the portal circulation after birth, there is a temporary diminution in liver volume. The next change is constriction of the sphincter at the entry into the ductus venosus so that all the blood reaching the liver must now pass through the liver sinusoids. The next phenomenon is closure of the foramen ovale and the mechanism by which this is brought about has already been described. This is followed by closure of the ductus arteriosus.

All of the changes that have been described are first of all functional changes. In other words, when the ductus arteriosus and the umbilical vessels close, they do so by vasoconstriction and the closure of the foramen ovale is brought about by apposition of the interatrial septa. Only later is there anatomical closure as a result of proliferation of the endothelium of the vessels concerned, which then undergo fibrosis. Similarly, there is a proliferation of fibrous tissue in between the septum primum and the septum secundum. As a result of these changes, various rudimentary structures of adult anatomy are produced. Thus the left umbilical vein forms the fibrous cord which connects the umbilicus to the porta hepatis of the liver, called the ligamentum teres (round ligament) of the liver and this joins the left branch of the portal vein at the porta hepatis (Fig. 79). The ductus venosus forms the ligamentum venosum. It is therefore obvious from Fig. 79 that if the ligamentum teres is followed along the free border of the falciform ligament in adult life, it will pass into the fissure for the ligamentum teres in the liver and then become continuous with the ligamentum venosum (in the fissure for the ligamentum venosum), which in turn is attached to the inferior vena cava.

When the foramen ovale closes, the fossa ovalis remains on the right side of the interatrial septum, indicating the site of this in the adult. The ductus arteriosus forms the ligamentum arteriosum and this connects the left pulmonary artery with the aorta just below the arch. The ligamentum arteriosum is, therefore, the remains of the continuation of the left sixth arch artery in fetal life. The nerve associated with the sixth pharyngeal arch is the recurrent laryngeal nerve and this curves around the ligamentum arteriosum in the adult (Fig. 73). On the right side, however, the corresponding part of the sixth arch artery disappears and, during "descent" of the heart, the right recurrent laryngeal nerve will only be stopped by the next arch artery with which it comes into contact and this is the fourth arch artery which, on the right side, forms the subclavian artery. The asymmetry in development of the arterial circulation therefore explains the difference in course of the recurrent laryngeal nerve on the two sides in the adult.

References

Ashworth, A. M. and Neligan, G. A. (1959). Changes in the systolic blood pressure of normal babies during the first twenty-four hours of life. *Lancet* **256,** 804-807.

Barclay, A. E., Franklin, K. J. and Pritchard, M. M. L. (1944). "The Foetal Circulation" Blackwell Scientific Publications, Oxford.

Born, G. V. R., Dawes, G. S., Mott, J. C. and Widdicombe, J. G. (1954). Changes in the heart and lungs at birth. *Cold Spring Harb. Symp. quant. Biol.* **19,** 102-108.

Gunther, M. (1957). The transfer of blood between baby and placenta in the minutes after birth. *Lancet* **252,** 1277-1280.

Lower, R. (1669). "Tractatus de Corde". Redmayne, London.

16

The Urogenital System

The development of nephric units

The urogenital system develops in, or in close association with, the intermediate mesoderm, which is that part of the intraembryonic mesoderm in between the paraxial mesoderm medially and the lateral plate mesoderm laterally. Because of the lateral flexion of the body wall, the intermediate mesoderm is carried into a more ventral position (Fig. 32) and forms a bulge on either side of the root of the mesentery; each bulge has a groove on either side of it, the lateral and medial coelomic bays. Just as with other aspects of development, so the development of the urogenital apparatus has been considered to recapitulate the embryonic history of the lower vertebrates. Thus, the most primitive adult vertebrate kidney, the *pronephros,* is first formed in human development from the intermediate mesoderm in the cervical region. It consists of excretory tubules which are so primitive that they are probably non-functional in man. The pronephros soon degenerates and the next most caudal part of the intermediate mesoderm from the lower cervical region to the lumbar region begins to differentiate into another primitive kidney called the mesonephros. The *mesonephros* also has excretory tubules (Fig. 34) which are functional and, while it differentiates into the adult kidney in amphibia, it only forms a temporary functional structure in human development; it is even more functional in the embryos of certain other mammals, for example the pig, and this can be correlated with the efficiency of the placenta (Bremer, 1916). Even the mesonephros, however, eventually degenerates and disappears as an excretory organ, but some of its tubules and its duct persist to form part of the male reproductive system and there are a few primitive embryonic remains in the female, which will be discussed later (pp. 167, 176). The mesonephros is replaced by a structure differentiated from the next most caudal part of the intermediate mesoderm which forms the definite human kidney or *metanephros.* Torrey (1954) has critically analysed this description of the succession of three kidney units and concludes that the concept of the pronephros does not apply to the human embryo. Further, there is a lack of clear-cut criteria by which one type of nephros may be distinguished from another, with particular reference to their cranio-caudal extent. He would prefer to consider these nephric units as intergrading regions of a *holonephros.*

The metanephros

Caudal to the pronephros a duct (the nephric duct) arises independently of the pronephric rudiment and passes down the dorsal (posterior) abdominal wall to open into the cloaca; when the mesonephros develops, it utilizes this duct for its own duct, which therefore becomes the *mesonephric* (*Wolffian*) *duct*. The metanephros develops in a slightly different fashion from two separate entities, the *metanephric cap* or *blastema* (Fig. 81), which differentiates from the intermediate mesoderm and the *ureteric bud* or *diverticulum* (Fig. 82), which is a diverticulum from the lower end of the mesonephric duct. The ureteric bud grows dorsolaterally from the meso-nephric duct just before the latter joins the cloaca, to meet the metanephric cap. The metanephric blastema develops caudal to the mesonephros and it must, therefore, differentiate in the intermediate mesoderm of the last two lumbar segments and the upper sacral segments. Just as the testis migrates downwards in its development, so also must the kidney later migrate upwards relatively in its development, owing to differential growth rates, to reach its adult position below the diaphragm. Since the metanephric kidney develops from two parts, the different components of the adult kidney have different origins. The metanephric blastema forms the majority of the adult kidney. In the nephron, which is the unit of the kidney structure, the metanephric blastema forms all of this unit in each case from Bowman's capsule down to the collecting tubules. The ureteric diverticulum forms the ureter, the renal pelvis the major and minor calyces and the collecting tubules.

Löfgren (1949), in an investigation of the development and structure of the human kidney, discovered that there are seven ventral and seven dorsal components each being composed of a branch of the renal pelvis with its corresponding pyramid and representing a fundamental embryonic unit. Grooves between each of the seven pairs of components are obvious on the surface of the kidney and persist throughout fetal life, so producing *fetal lobulation* of the kidney, which may be apparent even in adult life in some kidneys. The boundary between the ventral and dorsal components is also marked on the surface of the kidney by a longitudinal sulcus along its lateral border. Graves (1954, 1956) has shown that there are five branches of the renal artery within the kidney which supply corresponding segments of it; there is no collateral arterial circulation between the segments.

Development of the gonads

The reproductive system develops in close association with the urinary system. The mesonephros is covered on its abdominal surface by splanchno-pleuric intraembryonic mesoderm, which thickens on the medial aspect of the mesonephros in the medial coelomic bay to form a swelling (Fig. 33). This swelling, the *genital* (*gonadal*) *ridge* (Figs 83, 84) extends along the medial aspect of the mesonephros and then becomes condensed to approx-imately its middle two quarters. The primordial germ cells migrate into this gonadal ridge from the endoderm of the yolk sac (Witschi, 1948; Chiquoine, 1954) by passing dorsally through the mesenchyme in the root of the mesentery, and then *sex* (*rete*) *cords* (Figs 33, 85) proliferate in the substance of the gonadal ridge from the coelomic epithelium formed by the splanchno-pleuric intraembryonic mesoderm. Up to this stage, development is the same whether the gonad is to form a testis or an ovary. In the case of the testis, the sex cords persist and form the seminiferous tubules (Fig. 86) and rete testis (Fig. 87), but in the developing ovary, they break up and form a *degenerate rete ovarii.*

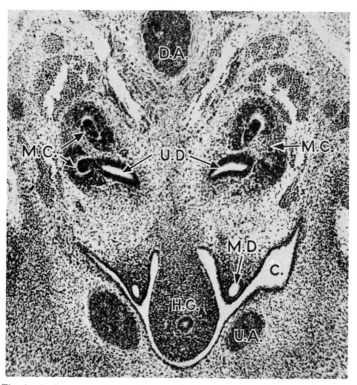

Fig. 81. The developing metanephroi of a 13 mm human embryo. The metanephric cap (M.C.) and ureteric diverticulum (U.D.) can be seen in each metanephros. The hindgut (H.G.) suspended by its mesentery in the coelom (C.) and bounded on each side by the mesonephric ducts (M.D.) are also visible. The dorsal aorta (D.A.) and umbilical arteries (U.A.) are present in this section also. ($\times$ 77).

Gillman (1948) claims that the coelomic epithelium of the gonadal ridge provides the granulosa cells of the ovary and (probably) the Sertoli cells in the testis; the theca cell is a modified stroma cell of mesenchymal origin. He confirms that the germ cells arise outside the gonad primordium.

The primitive gonad becomes separated from the mesonephros and in doing so forms a mesentery (Fig. 88), which in the case of the testis is called the *mesorchium* and in the ovary the *mesovarium.* Later there is an atrophy of the upper part of the gonadal ridge so that there is a relative descent of the gonad and then later a more complete descent to its definitive position. This

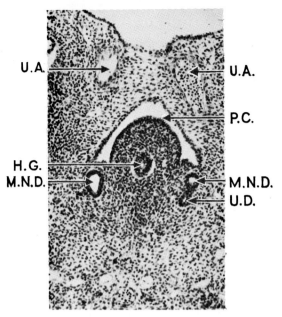

Fig. 82. The ureteric diverticulum (U.D.) arising from the mesonephric duct (M.N.D.) of a 7 mm human embryo. The hindgut (H.G.), peritoneal cavity (P.C.) and umbilical arteries (U.A.) may also be seen. (× 77).

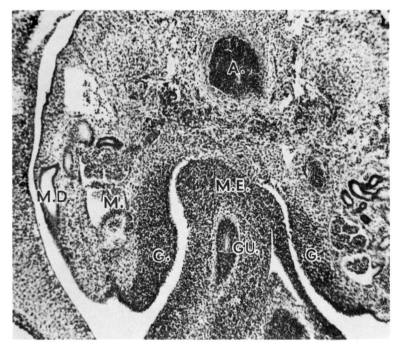

Fig. 83. A transverse section through the mesonephroi (M.) and gonadal ridges (G.) of a 13 mm human embryo. The dorsal aorta (A.), mesonephric duct (M.D.) and the gut (GU.) with its mesentery (M.E.) are also visible. (× 77).

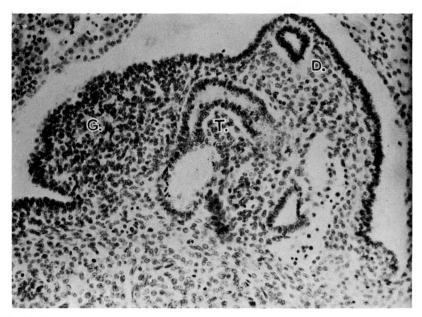

Fig. 84. The developing gonad (G.) in a 12·5 mm human embryo, formed as a swelling on the medial aspect of the mesonephros; one of the mesonephric tubules (T.) and the mesonephric duct (D.) are clearly visible. (From Giroud, 1958.)

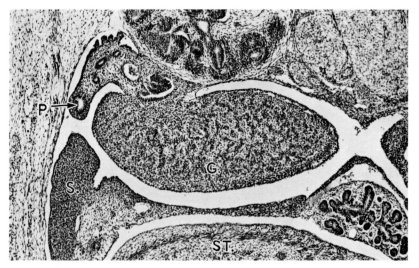

Fig. 85. The developing gonad (G.) in a 20 mm human embryo seen from the superior aspect in transverse section. The sex cords within the gonad are clearly visible. The spleen (S.), stomach (ST.) and paramesonephric duct (P.) can also be seen in this section. (From Giroud, 1958.)

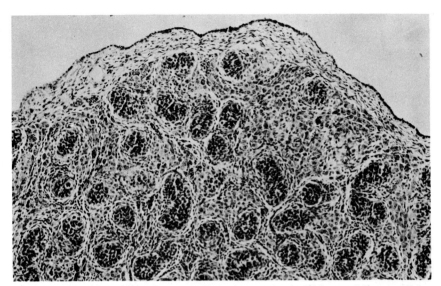

Fig. 86. The testis in a 4½-month human fetus showing the developing seminiferous tubules separated by large quantities of interstitial tissue. (From Giroud, 1958.)

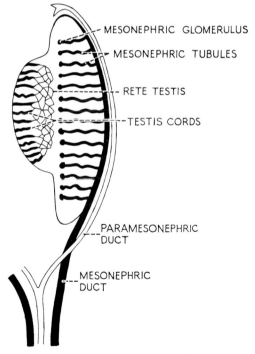

Fig. 87. The developing testis, seen from the ventral aspect. The sex cords have developed into the testis cords (which form the seminiferous tubules) and rete testis which must later join with the ductuli efferentes formed from the mesonephric tubules. (From Giroud, 1958.)

relative descent is caused by the rapid growth of the caudal part of the vertebral canal (see p. 194). The *gubernaculum testis,* a column of mesenchyme extending from the lower pole of the testis towards the developing scrotum, which was formerly thought to pull down the testis in its descent, is now known (Backhouse and Butler, 1960) to form the cremaster muscle. It guides the testis during descent and dilates the pathway. The gubernaculum is also

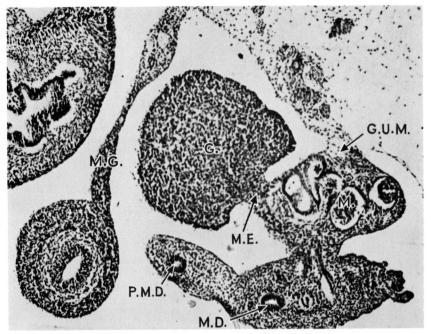

Fig. 88. The left gonad (G.), suspended by its mesentery (M.E.) from the medial aspect of the mesonephros (M.) of a 28·5 mm human embryo. The genito-urinary mesentery (G.U.M.), paramesonephric (P.M.D.) and mesonephric (M.D.) ducts are also visible. The gonad is lying in the medial coelomic bay, medial to the mesonephros and lateral to the mesentery of the gut (M.G.). (× 77).

the site of development of the *processus vaginalis,* a pouch of peritoneum which becomes invaginated by the testis. By the seventh month of fetal life, the testis commences to pass through the inguinal canal and normally reaches the scrotum at the eighth month or, at the latest, by the time of birth. The neck of the process vaginalis becomes obliterated soon after birth; only the lower part of the processus remains as the tunica vaginalis.

Development of gonadal duct systems

It must be stressed that the development of the gonad is identical to a certain stage in both sexes; in other words, an embryo is at first potentially bisexual and duct systems associated with the gonad develop identically in both sexes up to a certain stage. The duct system for the male is a pair of mesonephric (Wolffian) ducts and in the female a non-urinary structure, the paired paramesonephric (Müllerian) ducts. In both sexes both mesonephric and paramesonephric ducts develop and only in later development does one or other of them undergo predominance to form the duct system associated with the specific sex—the mesonephric ducts in the male and the paramesonephric ducts in the female. The paramesonephric duct is formed by an invagination of the coelomic epithelium (splanchnopleuric intraembryonic mesoderm) on the lateral, dorsolateral, ventrolateral or ventral surface (see Faulconer, 1951) of the mesonephros to form a tube. Although this gives rise to the accessory sex organs of the female, the uterine tubes, the uterus and the scaffolding of the vagina, it is present also in the male but never develops to the same extent as in the female. In the male, the ductus deferens and the epididymis are formed from the mesonephric duct and the rete testis develops from the sex cords inside the gonad (Figs 87, 89). These structures are connected with one another in the adult by the ductuli efferentes which differentiate from some of the mesonephric tubules (see Giroud, 1958). There are also a variety of rudimentary structures and tubules which are formed from the mesonephric tubules and duct. Thus, the ductuli aberrantes and paradidymis, rudimentary tubules associated with the epididymis, develop from the mesonephric tubules. From the mesonephric duct itself, apart from the ductus deferens and the epididymis, can arise the appendix epididymidis, a small cystic structure attached to the head of the epididymis. The mesonephric ducts also form the ejaculatory ducts and, as diverticula, the seminal vesicles.

The paramesonephric ducts, apart from developing into the *uterovaginal canal* in the female, in the male give rise to the appendix testis (hydatid of Morgagni), which is a small cystic structure very frequently attached to the superior pole of the testis. These ducts also form a rudimentary *uterus masculinus* or *prostatic utricle*, a diverticulum about half way along the posterior wall of the prostatic urethra. The lower end of the utricle is developed, together with the colliculus seminalis, from cells having origin in the endoderm of the urogenital sinus and mesodermal mesonephric duct cells, as well as paramesonephric duct cells (Glenister, 1962). The mesonephric tubules produce some rudimentary tubules lying in the broad ligament associated with the ovary called the paroophoron and epoophoron. The mesonephric duct itself may persist as a duct which passes medially in the broad ligament to the side of the uterus and there runs down the side of the uterus and the vagina as a rudimentary canal, the duct of Gärtner.

Sexual differentiation

The embryonic hormonal control of sexual differentiation in vertebrates has been analysed by Moore (1947). Whereas it is possible to produce modifications in the gonads of amphibia and other vertebrates by hormone treatment (see Dantschakoff, 1941) so that even complete sex inversion may occur, study of the development of the reproductive system of mammals has failed to contribute evidence supporting the hormone concept of gonadal differentiation. In the mammals, sex hormones can stimulate the growth of embryonic sex ducts; thus, administered oestrogenic hormones may cause the growth and differentiation of the paramesonephric ducts in a genetic male embryo. There is, however, no dependable evidence that hormones can modify the development of the gonad of a mammal. Further, in no vertebrate is there evidence that hormones are secreted by developing gonads during the

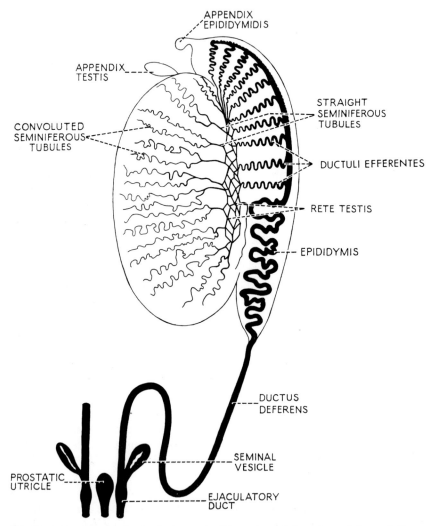

Fig. 89. A later stage in the developing testis. The testis cords have formed the seminiferous tubules and the epididymis has developed from the mesonephric duct. Some of the mesonephric tubules have developed into the ductuli efferentes (vasa efferentia). (From Giroud, 1958.)

period when the embryonic duct system undergoes modification into the definitive male or female type. In mammals, the evidence suggests that hormones are secreted by gonads during the latter part of gestation, after the development of the embryonic reproductive duct systems. The most acceptable evidence for the control of sex differentiation in mammals rests upon the operation of genetic sex differentiating factors unconnected with sex hormone actions.

Bladder and prostate gland

The bladder develops from the urogenital sinus which is the ventral half of the primitive cloaca after it has been divided by the urorectal septum (Figs 50, 90). The urogenital sinus first undergoes differential dilatation to form from below upwards a *pars phallica,* a *pars pelvina* and a *vesico-urethral canal* (Fig. 51) which is continuous at its apex with the allanto-enteric diverticulum. As its name suggests, the vesico-urethral canal develops into the bladder and the urethra; although it forms the whole of the urethra in the female it only produces the upper part of the prostatic urethra in the male. As can be seen from Fig. 51, the mesonephric duct empties into the urogenital sinus at the junction between the pars pelvina and the vesico-urethral canal. The mesonephric duct develops into the ejaculatory duct at its lower end and in the adult this opens into the prostatic urethra at approximately its mid-point; the vesico-urethral canal, therefore, only forms the upper part of the prostatic urethra, while the lower part of the prostatic urethra and the membranous urethra develop from the pars pelvina. This also has an important consequence in the development of the prostate. In the adult the median lobe of the prostate is found above the ejaculatory ducts; the remainder of the prostate consists of an anterior, a posterior and two lateral lobes, although the distinction between these different lobes is very difficult in the adult. The glands of the median lobe differ from those of the other lobes in developing from the epithelial cells of the colliculus seminalis. The glands of the other lobes, however, develop from four diverticula, anterior, posterior and two lateral, from the endoderm of the pars pelvina. These diverticula only form tubules from which develop the glands and ducts of the prostate; the connective tissue and muscular tissue develop from the mesoderm which surrounds them.

During the last months of fetal life, the epithelium of the tubules of the prostate shows squamous metaplasia, proliferation and alteration of the epithelium of the tubules, fully differentiated epithelium, dilatation of the tubules and hyperplasia; these changes persist for 1-4 weeks after birth and gradually regress over a period of 1-4 months, although the ejaculatory ducts remain dilated for longer (Andrews, 1951). In late fetal life it is difficult to distinguish the five fundamental lobes of the prostate (see Lowsley, 1930), and they become even less distinct in postnatal life, particularly the posterior lobe; the median lobe is always recognizable, however, since it is that part lying above the ejaculatory ducts, posterior to the urethra. At puberty the tubules develop into the prostatic glands and ducts, the majority of which open into the prostatic sinuses (Fig. 91) and are therefore concentrically arranged: a few smaller mucosal and submucosal glands, however, open into the anterior and posterior walls of the urethra.

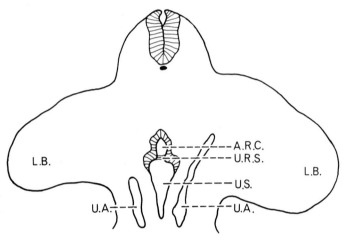

Fig. 90. The cloaca of a 6·5 mm human embryo showing its division by the urorectal septum (U.R.S.) into anorectal canal (A.R.C.) dorsally, and the urogenital sinus (U.S.) ventrally, which is closely related on either side to the umbilical arteries (U.A.). The limb buds (L.B.) are also visible. The neural groove is just on the point of closing to form the neural tube. Camera lucida drawing of histological section. (× 51).

Penis and urethra

The pars phallica forms the urethra inside the body (shaft) of the penis, including that in the glans penis (see Paul and Kanagasuntheram, 1956; Glenister, 1958). The endoderm of this part of the urogenital sinus first proliferates to form the *urethral plate*. This becomes flanked on each side by the genital folds (see p. 173) which, in the male, fuse together over the urogenital membrane to form the body of the penis when this membrane disintegrates, so converting the pars phallica into an open inverted trough lined with endoderm. The urethral plate also extends on to the lower aspect of the genital tubercle and here again becomes bounded on each side by the genital folds, so forming the primitive *urethral groove* which will, of course, be continuous with the trough formed from the pars phallica. After disintegration of epithelium in these structures the genital folds grow together and fuse, first over the open pars phallica and then progressively towards the tip of the glans over the urethral groove in such a way that only epithelium derived from the urethral plate or from the urogenital sinus is included in the lining of these parts of the urethra. The ectoderm lining the more superficial aspect of the genital folds when they fuse, may contribute to the floor of the glandar urethra (Kanagasuntheram and Anandaraja, 1960) and forms the perineal raphe. The terminal portion of the glandar urethra— the fossa navicularis and sinus of Guérin—develops from an ingrowth of ectoderm on the genital tubercle.

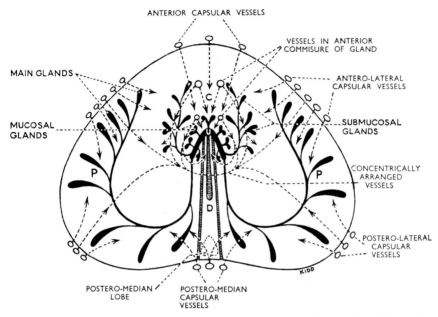

Fig. 91. Diagrammatic transverse section through the prostate showing the disposition of the blood vessels supplying it and the glands (P.) within its substance. The prostatic urethra (U.) has the colliculus seminalis along its posterior border, opening on the apex of which is the prostatic utricle (D.) with the ejaculatory ducts on either side of it. On either side of the colliculus, the ducts of the prostatic glands are seen opening into the prostatic sinuses. Modified from Clegg (1956).

In the female the pars phallica and the pars pelvina open up and form the vestibule and the whole of the urethra develops from the lower part of the vesico-urethral canal.

Vagina and uterus

The paramesonephric ducts fuse in their lower parts to produce a single tube called the uterovaginal canal. The lower end of this canal proliferates to form a tubercle called the Müllerian tubercle and this abuts on the upper part of the posterior wall of the pars pelvina. The whole of the uterovaginal canal lies in a transverse band of mesoderm, the *urogenital septum* (Fig. 92), continuous with the urorectal septum. Proliferations from the pars pelvina of the urogenital sinus grow up to form the epithelium lining the whole of the vagina (Bulmer, 1957). There is some experimental evidence to suggest that the vaginal epithelium in the mouse is formed in part from Müllerian tissue as well as from cells derived from the urogenital sinus (Forsberg, 1965). The unfused parts of the paramesonephric ducts develop into the uterine tubes; where they fuse together they form the uterovaginal canal, which develops into the uterus and acts as the scaffolding upon which the vagina is formed.

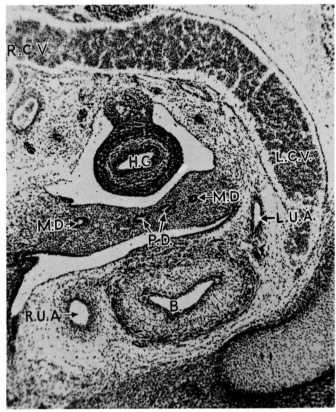

Fig. 92. Transverse section through the urogenital septum containing paramesonephric (P.D.) and mesonephric (M.D.) ducts in a 28·5 mm human embryo. The septum is lying in between hindgut (H.G.) and bladder (B.). The right (R.U.A.) and left (L.U.A.) umbilical arteries lie on each side of the bladder, and the right (R.C.V.) and left (L.C.V.) common iliac veins are visible. (× 52).

External genitalia

The proliferation of mesoderm that surrounds the lower end of the anal canal also continues to surround the lower end of the urogenital sinus and in doing so, helps to form the external genitalia; it also extends on to the ventral aspect of the urogenital sinus and here it forms the infraumbilical region of the body wall (Wyburn, 1937; Glenister, 1958). It can be seen from Fig. 51 that this mesoderm also forms the dorsal aspect of the body of the penis. Just as in the case of the gut, endoderm of the vesico-urethral canal only differentiates into the epithelium of the mucous membrane of the bladder. The muscle and connective tissue of the bladder are formed from the infra-umbilical mesoderm. The trigone of the bladder is formed differently from the remainder by developing from the portion of the lower end of the mesonephric ducts, between the site of the ureteric diverticulum and the opening of the ducts into the bladder, which becomes absorbed into the vesico-urethral canal. This process is responsible for the ejaculatory ducts and ureters coming to open separately into the urinary tract.

The proliferation of mesoderm which encircles the lower end of the urogenital sinus raises up two pairs of eminences (Fig. 93). The medial pair of eminences are called the genital folds while the lateral paired eminences are the *genital swellings*. The genital folds in the female form the labia minora, and the genital swellings the labia majora; the genital tubercle forms the clitoris. In the male, however, the genital folds fuse together to form the body of the penis, the genital tubercle forming the glans penis, while the genital swellings form the scrotum. The genital folds are sometimes called the urethral folds but this term is misleading because only in the male do they close over to form the urethra. Up to a certain stage of development, therefore, the embryo is also potentially bisexual as regards its external genitalia, since there is an indeterminate stage at which it is impossible to decide from examination of the external genitalia whether a male or a female will develop. In the male when the genital folds fuse together, there is a proliferation of cells so that the whole of the area beneath the genital folds, including the pars phallica, becomes solid and only later does this become re-canalized in order to form the urethra in the body of the penis. The urethra, once re-canalization has taken place, is therefore fundamentally composed in its posterior wall of endoderm and its anterior wall of ectoderm.

CLINICAL RELATIONSHIPS

Kidney abnormalities

Because of the complicated development of the kidney, several different abnormalities may occur. The kidney may fail to develop altogether, a condition which may be unilateral or bilateral and is called *renal agenesia;* when bilateral this is obviously incompatible with life. Unilateral renal agenesia is common, being found once in 552 post mortems; bilateral agenesia is five times less frequent. Infants with bilateral renal agenesia usually have a characteristic facial appearance—a flattened nose, receding chin, wide interpupillary distance and large, low-set ears (the "Potter facies"). In addition this condition may be accompanied by other abnormalities, such as fused lower extremities (syrenomelia) and oligamnios.

Unilateral renal agenesia is often asymptomatic and compatible with normal life span.

Since the kidney develops first of all in the pelvis and then ascends relatively, if it fails to do so a *congenital pelvic kidney* can result. This condition is almost invariably unilateral, often asymptomatic and occurs in about 0·1% persons. Very rarely the ascent continues and the kidney may be found

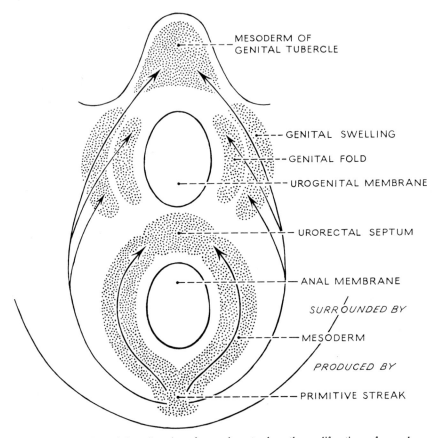

Fig. 93. Surface view of the tail region of an embryo to show the proliferations of mesoderm, shown in stipple, which lie underneath the ectoderm and surround the anal and urogenital membranes. The arrows show the direction of growth of the mesoderm and correspond to those shown in Fig. 51.

in an abnormally high condition, even intrathoracic, having ascended through a diaphragmatic defect. Ectopia of the kidney may occasionally (0·01-0·08% persons) manifest as "crossed" renal ectopia, when the kidney of one side lies on the opposite side, its ureter crossing the midline. Such a kidney may even fuse with its contralateral fellow, giving rise to a kidney with a bizarre shape. As the kidney "ascends" it changes its blood supply. It is therefore possible for the primitive arteries which supply the kidney during its ascent to persist. When this occurs, there are one or two aberrant renal arteries which arise either from the lower part of the aorta, inferior mesenteric artery, middle sacral artery, or from the common iliac artery (Bremer, 1915), and usually pass upwards to the kidney anterior to the ureter just below the pelvis and therefore compress the ureter (possibly intermittently). There is a resultant back pressure of urine in the ureter, and the pelvis and calyces dilate, a condition called hydronephrosis in which the renal pelvis and the calyces may become so ballooned out that the cortex of the kidney is merely a thin shell over the surface of this dilated bag of urine. Abnormalities in the number of renal arteries can occur. Although the usual pattern is for one artery to supply each kidney, Sykes (1964) found accessory renal arteries present in 25% kidneys, and when present supplied the kidney segment normally vascularized by either the apical or the lower segmental arteries.

Another abnormality which may occur results from malunion of the ureteric diverticulum and the metanephric blastema; the part of the nephron formed from the metanephric cap fails to unite with the collecting tubules formed from the ureteric diverticulum, so that a small cyst develops in this position. There may be a large number of cysts, a condition called polycystic kidney, or only a large single solitary cyst of the kidney. There are, however, other views regarding the origin of cystic disease of the kidney (see Willis, 1958). Polycystic kidney disease is very common, being found in one child in 265 to 450 post-mortems on children, and once in 222 to 1,019 adult post-mortems. It is almost invariably bilateral. The infantile form is fatal, death occurring within months after birth, while in adults the condition is progressive and recognized by the presence of pain resulting from progressively enlarging kidneys, haematuria, pyuria and eventually uraemia. Because of the differing characteristics of the infantile and adult forms of the disease, they must be considered as different diseases. The fact that the condition can persist into adult life is due to many of the cysts being "open", communicating at one pole with a patent collecting tubule or calyx, while all the cysts in the infantile type are closed. The anomaly is often associated with the presence of cysts in other organs (e.g. liver, pancreas, lung and spleen).

An interesting common abnormality is horseshoe kidney (found once in 425-1000 post-mortems) and the name describes exactly its appearance. The caudal ends of the metanephric blastemata are very close together and may rarely unite to form a kidney which has a horseshoe shape. Usually the ureteric diverticula in such cases are perfectly normal, so that the ureters issue normally from each side of the horseshoe kidney. About a third of such kidneys is usually perfectly normal in function and the anomaly is only discovered at post-mortem. Symptoms when present, consist of nausea, abdominal discomfort and pain on hyperextension (Rovsing syndrome) and may require surgical treatment. Irregular fusion of the bilateral metanephric blastemata may, more rarely, produce bizarre forms of kidney such as inverted horseshoe, V-shaped, "doughnut" and amorphous pelvic discoid or "lump" kidneys. The ureteric diverticulum is also subject to the formation of abnormalities. Normally when it reaches the metanephric blastema it starts to divide to form the calyces, but it can occasionally start to divide before reaching the metanephric cap, in which case a double ureter is formed. This condition is very common, occurring in 0·7-0·9% of all post-mortems, and is usually unilateral (85% cases) and asymptomatic in one-third of cases. In the other two-thirds, symptoms arise as a result of infection or obstruction of the urinary tract. The division of the ureter may be complete in 50% cases, each ureter having its own ureteric orifice into the bladder; in these cases two ureteric diverticula are formed instead of one on the affected side. Rarely the metanephric blastema may also divide in relation to each of the two diverticula, so producing a unilateral "double" kidney, or supernumerary kidney. In the 50% "incomplete" cases of double ureter, about 25% bifurcate in the distal third, 50% in the middle third and 25% in the proximal third of the ureter. There may be simply a bifid ureteric pelvis. Auer (1947) claims that the mesonephric duct has to be considered as the primary inductor of the mesonephros, ureter, kidney and Müllerian duct. It is interesting to note (see Hilson, 1957) that congenital anomalies of the urogenital system may be associated with deformities of the auricle.

Persistent rudimentary mesonephric tubules are of some importance because occasionally they enlarge pathologically and form cysts inside the broad ligament; when these cysts are small they are usually asymptomatic, but rarely a large cyst may be formed in the broad ligament which communicates with a patent duct of Gartner opening into the uterus or vagina or on the vestibule to one side of the orifice of the vagina. Such a large cyst may secrete a fluid which can be discharged along the duct to the exterior.

Hermaphroditism

The production of a true *hermaphrodite* has a genetic basis. In this rare condition the individual has gonads or gonadal tissue of both sexes. Thus, there may be an ovary on one side of the abdomen, and a testis on the other; or both gonads may be an ovotestis containing both ovarian and testis tissue. The external genitalia in a true hermaphrodite shows an admixture of both sexes; thus there may be both a vagina and a scrotum. Since the development of the scrotum, however, depends on the presence of testes, this may show varying degrees of development depending on whether the testes have descended or not. Butler *et al.* (1969) have shown that 53·5% of true hermaphrodites have a chromosome constitution similar to normal females (44XX), whilst the remainder are *mosaics* (in other words an admixture of chromosomal types, such as 44XX 44XY or 44XX 44XXY). A *pseudo-hermaphrodite* (having external genitalia of one sex, with gonads of opposite sex) may be caused by the action of hormonal factors operating from the suprarenal cortex; Wells and Wagenen (1954) have demonstrated that it is certainly possible to produce pseudohermaphroditism in the female rhesus monkey by introducing androgenic hormone into the maternal circulation during pregnancy, but failed to cause testicular changes in the gonads.

Generally, the disorder of the suprarenal cortex (see Chapter 22) which is associated with pseudohermaphroditism is hyperplasia (increase in the number of cells) which may be autonomous or occasioned by a basophil adenoma of the anterior lobe of the pituitary gland. The earlier in life that this hyperplasia occurs, the more severe the resultant disability. Thus, if it occurs during fetal life the hormonal imbalance causes a child with ovaries to be born with external genitalia which resemble the male, the clitoris being extremely enlarged, and the vagina diminutive or absent; similarly a fetus with testes will be born with hypospadias (vide infra) which may be so severe that the external genitalia resemble those in the female, and the testes have remained intra-abdominal in position. Even in later life such suprarenal cortical hyperplasia can produce virilism in adult women who show an enlargement of the clitoris and growth of hair on the face, or feminization in adult men.

Age changes in prostate

In late adult life the prostate may undergo one of several changes; it may atrophy, remain unchanged, or show pathological changes which, if they affect the glandular tissue, produce carcinoma, or, by proliferation of the connective tissue cause benign prostatic hyperplasia. Prostatic carcinoma is probably caused in most causes by enhanced androgenic activity and may be ameliorated or even cured by surgical castration; the same effect may also be achieved by action directly on the tumour cells or indirectly by "physiological castration" (probably caused by suppressing pituitary activity) after adminis-tration of large doses of oestrogens. Sensitivity to hormones varies from one part of the tumour to another (Franks, 1958), and this may be an indication of differing susceptibility of cells to the action of hormones. Prostatic hyperplasia occurs in response to a high oestrogen/androgen ratio in the body tissues.

Ectopia vesicae

Failure of fusion of the bilateral contributions of mesoderm which form the infra-umbilical region of the body wall results in a median cleft in this part of the anterior wall of the abdomen through which the bladder herniates once in 10,000 births (ectopia vesicae or exstrophy of the bladder). This same mesoderm also forms the connective tissue and muscle of the bladder wall. In some cases of ectopia vesicae, therefore, there may be a defect in the anterior wall of the bladder which may be laid open so that it is possible to see the orifices of the ureters opening into it. In the male, since this mesoderm also forms the dorsal aspect of the shaft of the penis, a minor degree of failure of fusion of the mesodermal contributions here will result in a defect in the dorsal aspect of the penis which allows the urethra to open to the exterior; such a condition is called epispadias. The process of fusion of the genital folds occurs from behind forwards and may fail to occur either in whole or in part; in the former case a cleft penis results, but in the latter case, usually occurring immediately behind the corona glandis, there is a small fistula which communicates the urethra with the exterior, a condition called hypospadias. In both hypospadias and epispadias urine escapes through the abnormal aperture, since the urethra in the glans may fail to develop properly.

Gonadal disorders

One or other or both gonads may fail to develop partially or completely in 0·04-0·5% persons when sexual infantilism results. A primary disorder of the hypothalamus or pituitary may have the same effect by withdrawing gonadotrophin control of the gonads, and results in such syndromes as Frohlich's syndrome (hypothalamic infantilism with obesity), and pituitary hypogonadism (hypopituitarism with dwarfism and sexual infantilism); in pure pituitary hypogonadism (pituitary eunuchoidism) there is a specific lack of pituitary gonadotrophic activity, not accompanied by dwarfism (Wilkins, 1966). In primary gonadal disorders, such as the ovarian agenesis seen in Turner's syndrome, the excretion of gonadotrophins may be increased, rather than decreased as in pituitary and hypothalamic hypogonadism. The gonadal dysgenesis in such cases may be so severe that the ovaries are merely represented by long white "streaks" in the broad ligaments; histologically such "streak gonads" are composed only of connective tissue with no obvious germ cells.

In Klinefelter's syndrome there is testicular dysgenesis. The external genitalia may be normal, but the testes are small and firm. The excretion of urinary gonadotrophins is increased. Unilateral absence of one testis (anorchia) is not uncommon, particularly in the cryptorchid person, but bilateral anorchia is rare.

Cryptorchidism

About 10% of newborn boys have undescended testes, but by puberty this figure is only about 0·5%. The cryptorchid testis must be distinguished from the retractile testis; in some boys an active cremasteric reflex causes the testis to be withdrawn into the inguinal canal, but it can be replaced in the scrotum following manipulation by the physician. In true cryptorchidism the testes remain in the abdomen (25%) or inguinal canal (75%), even after puberty, and only surgical intervention will enable them to be placed in the scrotum. Abdominally retained testes show a high incidence of tumours, some malignant, and may require removal; the higher temperature of the abdominal cavity causes eventual degeneration of the testes and spermato-genesis does not occur. The testis may also be found abnormally in an ectopic site; it has descended normally, but has been diverted by abnormal attachment of the gubernaculum testis into a femoral, perineal, pubopenile or superficial inguinal position. Since testicular descent is under hormonal control, administration of chorionic gonadotrophin prepubertally is often effective in ensuring descent in minor degrees of cryptorchidism.

The processus vaginalis, the pouch of peritoneum which accompanies the testis in its descent, may fail to be closed off to form a tunica vaginalis. In such a condition peritoneal fluid can accumulate in the processus, so forming a congenital hydrocele; or only a small part of the processus may remain to form an encysted hydrocele of the spermatic cord. A patent, persistent processus with a large neck will allow the herniation of abdominal contents through the inguinal canal into the sac formed by the processus—a congenital inguinal hernia.

Anomalies of the uterus and vagina

If the two paramesonephric ducts do not fuse together, varying degrees of duplication of the female reproductive tract may occur in 0·13-0·16% women. Complete duplication of the uterus and vagina occurs in monotremes and some marsupials, and since it occurs in the opossum *Didelphys virginiana,* it is therefore often described as uterus didelphys. The uterus only may be double, with a single vagina—uterus bicornis bicollis. In a bicornuate uterus, uterus bicornis unicollis, there is only one cervix, but two separate horns of the uterus. One of the uterine horns in such a case may be quite diminutive, and a mere appendage of the other horn, which has formed a uterus almost as complete as the normal. In bipartite uterus (uterus septus), the uterine cavity is divided by a median septum. Many of these variations in form of the uterus occur normally in some mammals. Thus the bicornuate uterus occurs in ungulates, and the bipartite uterus occurs in some carnivores.

Congenital absence of the uterus or vagina, or of the uterine tubes is usually associated with pseudohermaphroditism (p. 176). The hymen may remain imperforate and this may remain unnoticed until menstruation commences, when the vagina and hymen become distended with menstrual blood (haematocolpos). The lower 1/5 of the vagina may remain solid and uncanalized.

Urachus

The allanto-enteric diverticulum usually becomes completely obliterated and its connective tissue persists as a fibrous cord, the urachus, extending from the apex of the bladder to the umbilicus. It remains patent only once in 50,000-60,000 persons, but small urachal cysts, usually asymptomatic, have been found in about a third of all cadavers. A patent urachus, producing a urachal fistula, is made obvious by the appearance of urine at the umbilicus, and is treated by surgical excision. The urachus normally forms the median umbilical ligament.

References

Andrews, G. S. (1951). The histology of the human foetal and prepubertal prostates. *J. Anat.* **85**, 44-52.

Auer, J. (1947). Bilateral renal agenesia. *Anat. Rec.* **97**, 283-292.

Backhouse, K. M. and Butler, H. (1960). The gubernaculum testis of the pig (Sus scrofa). *J. Anat.* **94**, 107-120.

Bremer, J. L. (1915). The origin of the renal artery in mammals and its anomalies. *Am. J. Anat.* **18**, 179-200.

Bremer, J. L. (1916). The interrelations of the mesonophros, kidney and placenta in different classes of animals. *Am. J. Anat.* **19**, 179-205.

Bulmer, D. (1957). The development of the human vagina. *J. Anat.* **91**, 490-509.

Butler, L. J., Snodgrass, G. J. A. I., France, N. E., Russell, A. and Swain, V. A. J. (1969). True hermaphroditism or gonadal intersexuality. *Arch. Dis. Childh* **44**, 666-680.

Clegg, E. J. (1956). The vascular arrangements within the human prostate gland. *Br. J. Urol.* **28**, 428-435.

Chiquoine, A. D. (1954). The identification, origin and migration of primordial germ cells in the mouse embryo. *Anat. Rec.* **118**, 135-146.

Dantschakoff, V. (1941). "Der aufbau des Geschlechts beim hoheren Wirbeltier" Gustav Fischer, Jena.

Faulconer, R. J. (1951). Observations on the origin of the Mullerian groove in human embryos. *Contr. Embryol.* **34**, 159-166.

Forsberg, J.-G. (1965). An experimental approach to the problem of the derivation of the vaginal epithelium. *J. Embryol. exp. Morph.* **14**, 213-222.

Franks, L. M. (1958). Some comments on the long-term results of endocrine treatment of prostatic cancer. *Br. J. Urol.* **30**, 383-391.

Gillman, A. (1948). The development of the gonads in man, with a consideration of the role of fetal endocrines and the histogenesis of ovarian tumours. *Contr. Embryol.* **32**, 81-131.

Giroud, A. (1958). "La Fonction Spermatogenetique du Testicule" p. 25. Masson, Paris.

Glenister, T. W. (1958). A correlation of the normal and abnormal development of the penile urethra and of the infra-umbilical abdominal wall. *Br. J. Urol.* **30**, 117-126.

Glenister, T. W. (1962). The development of the utricle and of the so-called "middle" or "median" lobe of the human prostate. *J. Anat.* **96**, 443-445.

Graves, F. T. (1954). The anatomy of the intrarenal arteries and its application to segmental resections of the kidney. *Br. J. Surg.* **42**, 132.

Graves, F. T. (1956). The anatomy of the intrarenal arteries in health and disease. *Br. J. Surg.* **43**, 605.

Hilson, D. (1957). Malformation of ears as sign of malformation of genito-urinary tract. *Br. med. J.* **ii**, 785-789.

Kanagasuntheram, R. and Anandaraja, S. (1960). Development of the terminal urethra and prepuce in the dog. *J. Anat.* **94**, 121-129.

Löfgren, F. (1949). "Das Topographische System der Malpighischen pyramiden der Menschenniere" A.-B. Gleerupska Univ.-Bokhandeln, Lund.

Lowsley, O. S. (1930). Embryology, anatomy and surgery of the prostate gland. *Am. J. Surg.* **8**, 526-541.

Moore, C. R. (1947). "Embryonic Sex Hormones and Sexual Differentiation" Charles C. Thomas, Springfield.

Paul, M. and Kanagasuntheram, R. (1956). The congenital anomalies of the lower urinary tract. *Br. J. Urol.* **28**, 118-125.

Sykes, D. (1964). Some aspects of the blood supply of the human kidney. *Symp. Zool. Soc. Lond.*, No. 11, pp. 49-56.

Torrey, T. W. (1954). The early development of the human nephros. *Contr. Embryol.* **35,** 175-197.

Wells, L. J. and Wagenen, G. van (1954). Androgen—induced female pseudo-hermaphroditism in the monkey (Macaca mulatta): anatomy of the reproductive organs. *Contr. Embryol.* **35,** 93-108.

Wilkins, L. (1966). "The Diagnosis and Treatment of Endocrine Disorders in Childhood and Adolescence" 3rd. Edn. Thomas, Springfield.

Willis, R. A. (1958). "The Borderland of Embryology and Pathology" Butterworths, London.

Witschi, E. (1948). Migration of the germ cells of human embryos from the yolk sac to the primitive gonadal folds. *Contr. Embryol.* **32,** 67-80.

Wyburn, G. M. (1937). The development of the infra-umbilical portion of the abdominal wall, with remarks on the aetiology of ectopia vesicae. *J. Anat.* **71,** 201-230.

17

The Histogenesis of Nerve Tissue

The neural tube

At the time of lateral flexion of the embryonic plate, there is a thickening of the ectoderm immediately overlying the notochord to form the *neural (medullary) plate*. The notochord is in the axial region of the embryo and is flanked on either side by the paraxial mesoderm; the two together constitute the *chorda-mesoderm field* of organizer action, which induces the overlying ectoderm to differentiate into the neural plate, which rises up at its lateral margins in order to form the neural folds (Figs 18, 20); these eventually approximate to one another (Fig. 90), fuse and the somatic ectoderm is reconstituted over the surface of the resultant *neural tube*. The rudiment of the neural plate is in turn necessary for the further differentiation of paraxial mesoderm. When the neural tube has developed, lying ventral to it, in order, are the notochord, dorsal aorta and root of the mesentery (Figs 32, 33). In its definite form its dorsal and ventral aspects are very thin and are called the roof and floor plates respectively; the lateral walls of the neural tube are very much thicker. The walls of the neural tube are one cell thick, the cells being tall and columnar with nuclei situated towards the lumen side of the cell. The lumen of the neural tube becomes the central canal of the spinal cord and ventricles of the brain. The cells composing the neural tube are the *primitive medullary epithelial cells,* from which almost all cells in the future central nervous system are developed, including the nerve cells, which in turn send out processes into the periphery away from the central nervous system.

Cytodifferentiation in neural tube

Because of the important clinical and pathological implications of the process, it is necessary to describe the histogenesis of cells inside the central nervous system from the primitive medullary epithelial cells. The first thing that may occur in such a cell is that the nucleus, instead of being situated towards the lumen, shifts into approximately the middle of the cell, so that it becomes spindle-shaped and is now called a *spongioblast.* The spongioblast becomes transformed into an *astrocytoblast,* which in turn is transformed into an *astrocyte,* a particular type of neuroglial cell which, as well as possessing the ordinary characteristics of such cells, i.e. support, was formerly thought to aid in the nutrition of the central nervous system tissue by transferring material from blood vessels into the central nervous system by one of its processes attached to the wall of an adjacent blood vessel. It is now known that astrocytes constitute a three dimensional network of cell bodies and radiating processes in which nerve cells and cerebral capillaries are embedded, a relationship very similar to spermatogenic cells and Sertoli cells. Fibrous astrocytes are responsible for scarring, the repair of central nervous tissue following injury, and are found primarily in the white matter. Protoplasmic astrocytes are found chiefly in grey matter. The cytoplasm of a medullary epithelial cell may shrink away from the periphery of the neural tube and become confined to the nucleus at the lumen side of the tube; such a cell has one of two possible fates. Either it forms a cell lining the cavities of the central nervous system, a strictly epithelial cell which undergoes no further mitotic division and is called an *ependymal cell,* or it forms a cell which has intense mitotic activity and is called a *germinal cell.* The germinal cell in turn may either form a *medulloblast* which can differentiate into an astrocyte or an *oligodendrocyte,* or it may differentiate into neuroblasts. The astrocyte has already been considered; the interfascicular oligodendrocyte is a cell with very special properties because, although it is quite small and has few short processes, it is responsible for the productionof myelin around the axons of nerve fibres of the central nervous system (see Bensted *et al.,* 1957). Perineuronal oligodendrocytes surround the cell bodies of neurones as satellite cells, while perivascular oligodendrocytes are to be found in the vicinity of blood vessels; these two types of neuroglial cell have also therefore been implicated in the nutrition of neuronal tissue.

When the germinal cells form neuroblasts they first of all differentiate into cells which have no processes and are therefore called apolar neuroblasts; such cells then push out two processes at diametrically opposite poles of the cell to become bipolar neuroblasts and then lose one of these processes to become unipolar neuroblasts. Finally, at the opposite end of the cell to the single process, several processes are pushed out as dendrites, so forming the multipolar neuroblast which is now clearly similar to an adult neuron; the original single process grows very considerably and forms the axon of the neuron. The region of the formation of these neuroblasts is mainly the ventral aspect of the neural tube which begins to bulge on either side so that the shape of the tube changes; the central canal is compressed ventrally to become "coffin shaped" in cross-section (Figs 94, 95).

The final type of neuroglial cell to develop in the neural tube, the microglial cell, is quite late in its appearance and only really begins to appear when blood vessels grow into the neural tube; it develops from the adventitia of the blood vessels and is therefore mesodermal in origin in contradistinction to all the other types of neuroglial cell which, as has been seen, are ectodermal in origin. Penfield (1932) described these cells as developing in the nervous system as "fountains" of microglia budding off from blood vessels growing into certain regions of the neural tube. Microglial cells act as scavengers of the central nervous system being able to phagocytose products of the disintegration of neurones following injury. Because the central canal soon takes on a coffin shape in cross-section there is a lateral sulcus in the neural tube called the *sulcus limitans* (Figs 34, 94), which divides the lateral wall into two zones, one dorsal to the sulcus which is called the *alar lamina* and one ventral to it called the *basal lamina,* these are sensory and motor in function, respectively. It has already been noted that neuroblasts first congregate particularly in the basal lamina which becomes motor in function; they send out their axonal processes towards the periphery as motor nerve fibres and so form the ventral root of the spinal nerve.

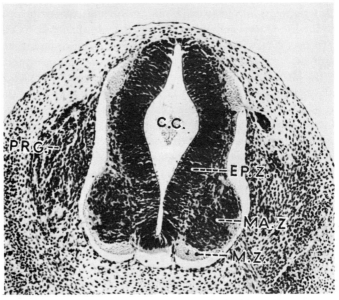

Fig. 94. Oblique transverse section through the developing neural tube of a 7 mm human embryo. The central canal (C.C.) is "coffin-shaped", and the ependymal (EP.Z.), mantle (MA.Z.) and marginal (M.Z.) zones are visible. The right dorsal root ganglion (P.R.G.) is also visible. (× 77).

Neural crest

Coincidental with cell proliferation and histogenesis in the neural tube there is some cell degeneration (Källén, 1955) which is localized to certain centres in early development but later becomes more generalized. This may be explained, in part by the regression and breakdown of those neuroblasts whose nerve fibres are not adequately sustained at the periphery (see Hamburger, 1958). The dorsal root ganglia and dorsal roots of the spinal nerves are derived from a tissue which is formed outside the central nervous system called the *neural crest,* which comes into being at the moment of fusion of the neural folds to produce the neural tube. Some of the cells at the site of fusion are left behind and remain dorsolateral to the neural tube and therefore outside it. The specialized strip of neural crest cells produced in this manner is in a convenient position for the development of dorsal root ganglion cells and their processes. These cells are first of all bipolar; the two processes then approximate to each other, fuse and therefore form a pseudo-unipolar cell which is the dorsal root ganglion cell. The process of the cell which grows out to the periphery is the dendrite of the cell, whereas that which grows into the central nervous system is the axon and is therefore much shorter than the dendrite.

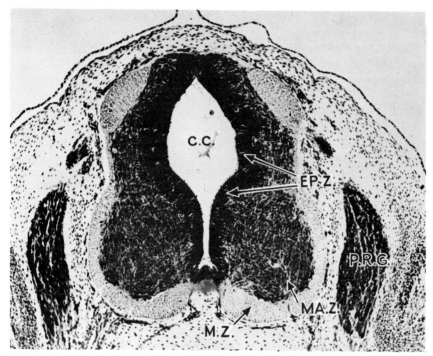

Fig. 95. The neural tube of a 13 mm human embryo. The central canal (C.C.) is beginning to close ventrally by proliferation of the mantle zone (MA.Z.) cells. The ependymal zone (EP.Z.) and marginal zone (M.Z.) and dorsal root ganglia (P.R.G.) are also visible. (× 77).

The dorsal root ganglion cell and its processes is therefore formed outside the central nervous system (Fig. 96) and when it connects with the central nervous system it does so secondarily. Since these peripheral nerve fibres develop outside the central nervous system, they cannot obtain their myelin from oligodendrocytes and therefore it must be produced from some other source, most probably the neurilemmal cells (Schwann cells) which are also of neural crest origin (see Causey, 1960). For this same reason there are no neurilemmal cells inside the central nervous system. Brizee (1949), however, has claimed that while the supporting cells of the spinal ganglia in the chick embryo are derived from neural crest, those of sympathetic ganglia are derived from indifferent cells some of which migrate from spinal ganglia via dorsal nerve roots, others migrate from the neural tube via ventral nerve roots; most of the supporting cells appear identical with oligodendrocytes but some develop into neurilemmal cells.

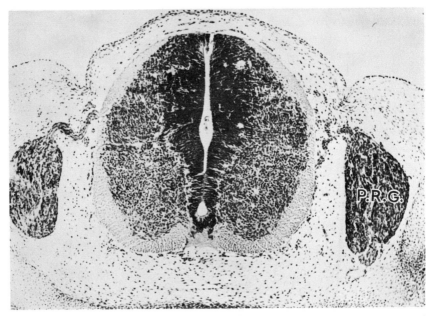

Fig. 96. Transverse section through the neural tube of a 17·5 mm human embryo. The shape of the central canal has altered, and fusion of its walls ventrally may be observed. The dorsal roots and their ganglia (P.R.G.) are clearly visible. ($\times$ 77).

Although the myelin inside the central nervous system and outside it is formed from different sources it seems to have the same chemical composition; as a result of X-ray diffraction studies it was found (Schmitt and Bear, 1939) that there are alternate layers of phospholipid and protein in the myelin sheath (see Causey, 1960), and the researches of Geren (1954) and Robertson (1955) indicate that these layers are arranged in the form of a spiral, and that a similar disposition is effected both inside and outside the central nervous system. A peripheral nerve fibre whenever it is cut or damaged, is able to regenerate, whereas a nerve fibre in the central nervous system does so with considerable difficulty, if at all (see Windle, 1956). Central nervous system neurons usually die when the axon is cut close to the cell body or if many axons are cut simultaneously; axonal sprouts from neurons that survive seem to be unable to reach or establish synaptic connexions.

In the regeneration of peripheral nerve fibres the neurilemmal cells play a very important part; such cells are absent inside the central nervous system and this may be responsible for its poor regenerative powers, in addition to the problem of neuroglial proliferation (see p. 238). Hogue (1950) has demonstrated that nerve cells and glia cells from the brains of fetuses and stillborn infants do not die when the individual dies. They can remain alive for long periods of time in refrigerated brain tissue and subsequently exhibit phenomena of growth in tissue culture.

As a result of the histogenesis of the various cells inside the neural tube it is possible to recognize three fundamental zones therein (Figs 94-97). Next to the lumen of the central canal are the ependymal cells which lie in the

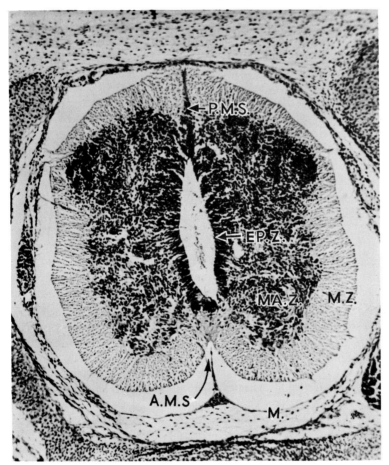

Fig. 97. A transverse section through the developing neural tube of a 28·5 mm human embryo, around which the meninges (M.) can be seen. Growth of the mantle zone (MA.Z.) in a ventral direction has brought into being the anteromedian sulcus (A.M.S.), while growth of the tube dorsally has obliterated the central canal here and produced the posteromedian septum (P.M.S.). The ependymal zone (EP.Z.) and marginal zone (M.Z.) are also visible. (× 77).

ependymal zone, while outside this are the neuroblasts and neuroglia which together constitute the *mantle zone;* outside this is the zone relatively free of cells into which nerve fibres grow and which is called the *marginal zone.*

It was suggested at one time by Ariens Kappers that a nerve fibre only becomes functionally active when it becomes myelinated. Langworthy (1929) showed that this is quite untrue, since some fibres can be myelinated and yet not be functional, while others are functional although not yet myelinated; he did, however, demonstrate that it is essential for a nerve fibre to become myelinated before it can participate in reflex activity.

Rexed (1944) has examined the nerve fibre size in the newborn and found that all motor cranial nerves and ventral roots show approximately the same degree of development. The calibre spectrum has a peak at 3-5μ, whereas the peak in dorsal roots is at 2-3μ. The regional differences between the spinal roots, so pronounced in adults, are scarcely indicated at birth and therefore develop in postnatal life.

Flechsig (1876) described areas of the cerebral cortex connected with specific nerve tracts according to the time when they become myelinated, because he thought that this would be related to the functional activity of the cerebral cortex. Since, however, myelination is not related absolutely to function, these *myelinogenetic areas* are not of any great value. Brodmann's cytoarchitectonic areas of the cerebral cortex (Brodmann, 1909; von Economo, 1929), however, are of great importance because the histological appearance of cells in the cerebral cortex is very closely related to its function.

In addition to the structures already mentioned it is known that the sympathetic nervous system and all chromaffin tissue, including the medulla of the suprarenal gland, develop from the neural crest (Hammond and Yntema, 1947; Hammond, 1949). The meninges around the spinal medulla develop from paraxial mesoderm; some cells from the neural crest mingle with these mesodermal cells and are primarily involved in forming the pia mater (Sensenig, 1951). The sensory ganglia associated with cranial nerves V, VII, IX and X are also formed from the neural crest (see Halley, 1955) but there is, in addition, a contribution to these ganglia from placodes, thickenings of ectoderm overlying their site of origin (Batten, 1957a, b and c). It has even been suggested that the optic cup which develops into a large part of the eye is also formed from the same source. There is a great deal of evidence also that melanoblasts develop from the neural crest (see Rawles, 1953; Niu, 1954, 1959) and the mesoderm of the pharyngeal arches has an origin from neural crest tissue (Horstadius, 1950).

CLINICAL RELATIONSHIPS

Defective closure of the neural tube leads to a flattened, open spinal cord—a persistence of the embryonic condition (myeloschisis). Such a condition is associated with spina bifida, and the defective spinal cord is contained in a sac which protrudes through the vertebral defect. The sac may contain only meninges (a meningocele) and when it contains the spinal cord as well it is termed a meningomyelocele. This condition occurs most frequently in the lumbosacral region, when the spinal cord may retain its length in the fetus, extending the whole length of the vertebral canal. In myelodysplasia there is a less severe but nevertheless incomplete closure of the neural tube. Rarely the central canal may have closed, but becomes dilated—the condition of syringomyelocele.

Variation in plexuses

As might be expected, there is considerable variation in the contribution of spinal nerves to the various plexuses. This is commonly seen in the brachial plexus when the deviations depend upon alterations in the level at which the various parts of the plexus separate and unite. Thus there may be only two cords in the plexus, one of them representing the union of two cords. The seventh cervical nerve sometimes divides into three branches, one passing to each of the cords. The ulnar nerve often (50% cases) has a contribution from the seventh cervical nerve, or may be formed wholly from the eighth nerve. It often gives off a branch to join the median, or vice versa. A very frequent anomaly is the variation in the level at which the two roots of the median nerve join: they may remain ununited until they have reached the level of the elbow. Similar variations may occur in the lumbosacral plexus, although less frequently. In both plexuses, a common variation is for the plexus to be prefixed or postfixed; the plexus as a whole arises from a slightly higher or lower level relative to the vertebral column than in the usually accepted position. Thus, in the prefixed brachial plexus ($\frac{2}{3}$ of all plexuses), a major part of the 4th cervical nerve joins the plexus (a branch from T_2 often being absent), while in the postfixed condition ($\frac{1}{3}$ of all plexuses) the 2nd thoracic nerve joins on to the first, within the thorax; the contributions from C4 being very small or completely absent. These can therefore be considered as "normal" variations. Such variations are obviously related to modifications in the migration, splitting and combination of the mesoderm which develops into the voluntary muscles of the limb.

Neuron variation

Large neurons (and usually the functions with which they are concerned) develop before small neurons. Neurons develop before neuroglia, and the time relationships differ in different parts of the nervous system and also in different mammals. There is some evidence to suggest that synapses are formed, and may even disappear, in response to functional demand.

The neurons in very young mammals (e.g. young rabbits and cats 8-15 days old) react differently to those in adults in the type of retrograde cell degeneration following damage to their axons. In one to two weeks after the damage all the cells disintegrate completely. This is the principle of the modified Gudden method used for studying experimentally the origin of certain nerve fibres.

Intermediate ganglia

Sympathetic ganglia may form in positions other than that accepted as normal. Such intermediate ganglia may be found attached to the ventral nerve roots, one or other ramus communicans (usually the grey rami communicantes in the cervical and lower lumbar regions) or to the trunks of the spinal nerves. The number of sympathetic ganglia varies considerably, since they have evolved in man by fusion between ganglia. The most primitive vertebrate condition was for the association of a single ganglion with one spinal nerve. As may be expected, therefore, there may be more or fewer sympathetic ganglia than normal. Thus, the middle cervical ganglion is often absent, fused with the superior ganglion, or represented by two ganglia.

Tumours

The pattern of histogenesis of the neural tube is of importance because tumours of the central nervous system often contain cells which have reverted to an embryonic type. Thus, whenever a glioma (a tumour of neurological origin) forms inside the central nervous system, its cells may revert to a more embryonic type, so that while it is possible for an astrocytoma to be formed from the adult astrocyte, an astrocytoblastoma can also develop and similarly a medulloblastoma or spongioblastoma may form (see Bailey, 1933).

References

Bailey, P. (1933). "Intracranial Tumours" Charles C. Thomas, Springfield.

Batten, E. H. (1957a). The activity of the trigeminal placode in the sheep embryo. *J. Anat.* **91,** 174-187.

Batten, E. H. (1957b). The epibranchial placode of the vagus nerve in the sheep. *J. Anat.* **91,** 471-489.

Batten, E. H. (1957c). The behaviour of the epibranchial placode of the facial nerve in the sheep. *J. comp. Neurol.* **108,** 393, 420.

Bensted, J. P. M., Dobbing, J., Morgan, R. S., Reid, R. T. W., and Payling Wright, G. (1957). Neurological development and myelination in the spinal cord of the chick embryo. *J. Embryol. exp. Morph.* **5,** 428-437.

Brizee, K. R. (1949). Histogenesis of the supporting tissue in the spinal and the sympathetic trunk ganglia in the chick. *J. comp. Neurol.* **91,** 129-146.

Brodmann, K. (1909). "Vergleichende Localisationslehre der Grosshirnrinde in ihren Prinzipien dargestellt auf Grund des Zellenbaues" Barth, Leipzig.

Causey, G. (1960). "The Cell of Schwann" E. & S. Livingstone, Edinburgh, London.

Economo, C. Von (1929). "The Cytoarchitectonics of the Human Cerebral Cortex" Oxford Univ. Press.

Flechsig, P. E. (1876). "Die Leitungsbahnen im Gehirn und Ruckenmark des Menschen" Engelmann, Leipzig.

Geren, B. B. (1954). The formation from the Schwann cell surface of myelin in the peripheral nerves of chick embros. *Exp. Cell Res.* **7,** 558-562.

Halley, G. (1955). The placodal relations of the neural crest in the domestic cat. *J. Anat.* **89,** 133-152.

Hamburger, V. (1958). Regression versus peripheral control of differentiation in motor hypo-plasia. *Am. J. Anat.* **102,** 365-410.

Hammond, W. C. (1949). Formation of the sympathetic nervous system in the trunk of the chick embryo following removal of the thoracic neural tube. *J. comp. Neurol.* **91,** 67-86.

Hammond, W. C., and Yntema, C. L. (1947). Depletions in the thoraco-lumbar sympathetic system following removal of neural crest in the chick. *J. comp. Neurol.* **91,** 67-86.

Hogue, M. J. (1950). Brain cells from human fetuses and infants, cultured in vitro after death of the individuals. *Anat. Rec.* **108,** 457-476.

Horstadius, S. (1950). "The Neural Crest" Oxford Univ. Press.

Källén, B. (1955). Cell degeneration during normal ontogenesis of the rabbit brain. *J. Anat.* **89,** 153-161.

Langworthy, O. R. (1929). A correlated study of the development of reflex activity in fetal and young kittens and the myelinization of tracts in the nervous system. *Contr. Embryol.* **20,** 127-174.

Niu, M. C. (1954). Further studies on the origin of amphibian pigment cells. *J. exp. Zool.* **125,** 199-220.

Niu, M. C. (1959). *In* "Pigment Cell Growth" ed. M. Gordon. p. 37. Academic Press, New York.

Penfield, W. (1932). *In* "Special Cytology" ed. E. V. Cowdry, 2nd. Edn., Chap. 36, p. 1445. Hoeber, New York.

Rawles, M. E. (1953). *In* "Pigment Cell Growth" ed. M. Gordon. p. 1. Academic Press, New York.

Rexed, B. (1944). Contributions to the knowledge of the postnatal development of the peripheral nervous system in man. *Acta psychiat. neurol. scand.* Suppl. **33,** 1-206.

Robertson, J. D. (1955). The ultrastructure of adult vertebrate peripheral myelinated nerve fibres in relation to myelinogenesis. *J. biophys. biochem. Cytol.* **1,** 271-278.

Schmitt, F. O. and Bear, R. S. (1939). The ultrastructure of the nerve axon sheath. *Biol. Rev.* **14,** 27-50.

Sensenig, E. C. (1951). The early development of the meninges of the spinal cord in human embryos. *Contr. Embryol.* **34,** 145-157.

Windle, W. F. (1956). Regeneration of axons in the vertebrate central nervous system. *Physiol. Rev.* **36,** 427-440.

18

Morphogenesis of the Neural Tube

The manner in which the neural tube comes to take the shape of the adult spinal cord is related to the fate of the tissue inside the neural tube. The neuroblasts congregate particularly in the basal lamina and in so doing, compress and eventually obliterate the ventral part of the central canal (Fig. 96). Since they proliferate ventrally they bulge on either side of the midline and so produce an *antero-median sulcus* (Figs 43, 97). Neuroblasts and neuroglia also proliferate in the alar lamina and similarly compress the central canal and obliterate it to produce the *postero-median septum* (Fig. 97). As a result, the central canal becomes very much constricted and occupies approximately the centre of the neural tube which thereby comes to take the form of the adult spinal cord. Only in the most caudal part of the neural tube which forms spinal cord, does the central canal not undergo reduction in size; it persists as a small dilatation called the *ventriculus terminalis* (Fig. 49).

Neuroblasts in the lateral walls of the spinal cord become arranged into columns (Fig. 98). One column in the alar lamina is concerned with the reception of afferent impulses from the periphery and is therefore called the *somatic afferent column* of neuroblasts. A collection of motor neuroblasts in the basal lamina similarly forms a *somatic efferent column*. Between the first thoracic and second or third lumbar segments two further columns of neuroblasts congregate around the sulcus limitans. These are associated with the sympathetic nervous system; the group of nerve cells immediately dorsal to the sulcus is called the *splanchnic (visceral) afferent column* of nerve cells, while that immediately ventral to the sulcus is called the *splanchnic (visceral) efferent column*. These columns are also associated with the parasympathetic nervous system in the 2nd to 4th sacral segments of the spinal cord.

This division of the neural tube by the sulcus limitans into motor (basal) and sensory (alar) components is related to the Bell law which states that there are two fundamental categories of nerves, namely motor and sensory. The most cephalic end of the neural tube develops into the brain and there has been some discussion as to how far forward this fundamental division of the neural tube can be considered to extend—i.e. how far forwards the sulcus limitans extends and it has been argued that it probably does so no further than the mid-brain, since the fore-brain is predominantly sensory in function and has no motor component. Since the hypothalamus is concerned predominantly with involuntary motor functions, however, it has been argued that the sulcus limitans extends forward as the sulcus between thalamus and

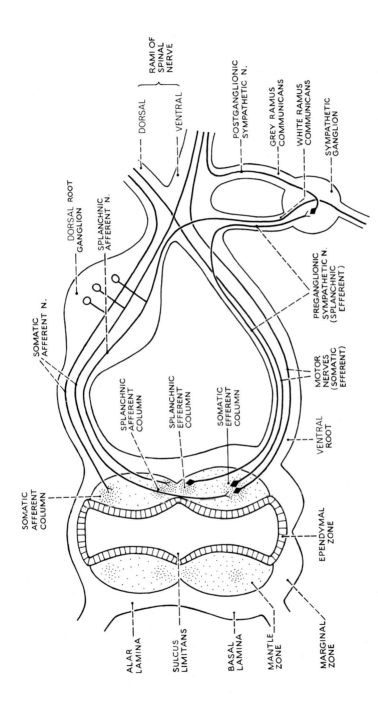

Fig. 98. Diagrammatic representation of a transverse section through the neural tube showing the cell columns in the mantle zone and the nerve fibres ending in relation to them.

hypothalamus. It is also possible to divide the neural tube transversely into elements called *neuromeres,* caused by waves of proliferation intensification within the neural tube (Bergquist and Källén, 1954), a process similar to metamerism in the paraxial mesoderm (Neal, 1918). In the spinal cord, the neuromeres are easily demarcated since each one corresponds to a segment of the spinal cord with its own spinal motor and sensory nerve. In the region of the hind-brain, this division is even more prominent, because here there are sulci which separate the neuromeres one from another; further forwards than this in the developing brain; however, it is not possible to demarcate them.

Differential growth rates

By the second month of fetal life the spinal cord is well formed and has spinal nerves attached to it; it extends the whole length of the vertebral canal. Its relationship to the vertebral column is not maintained, however, since the latter grows more rapidly than the neural tube. As a result it lags behind in development and its termination comes to lie at a relatively higher level (Fig. 99). Thus, shortly after the third month of fetal life, the caudal end of the spinal cord lies at the level of the first sacral vertebra. Although the dura mater extends the whole length of the vertebral column throughout life, the other meninges do not. Thus the pia mater, which closely invests the spinal cord, becomes pulled out from its tip as a long thread, the *filum terminale* (see Streeter, 1919), which extends therefore from the caudal end of the spinal cord down to the last coccygeal vertebra and may terminate there in a small cyst termed a *vestigeal coccygeal cyst.* This cyst, together with any primitive streak cells which may remain at the tail end of the embryo (Fig. 49) and probably also together with any post-coccygeal nerves which may persist, are usually shed with the atrophy of the tail.

The arachnoid mater does not retract so markedly in its relation to the vertebral column; in the adult it usually terminates at the level of the third sacral vertebra. The rate of "ascent" of the conus medullaris has been shown by Barson (1970) to be most rapid before the 17th week of gestation, when its level is opposite the fourth lumbar vertebra. There is a normal variation in the level of termination at any particular age and after the 17th week there is a much greater decline in growth rate, so that by birth the spinal cord terminates at the lower border of the second lumbar vertebra. By the second month, postnatally, the conus medullaris attains the "adult" level—at the lower border of the first lumbar vertebra or the upper border of the second lumbar vertebra. An important clinical consequence of this feature is that there is a portion of the subarachnoid space containing cerebrospinal fluid between L1 and S3 from which C.S.F. can be removed by the insertion of a needle between the laminae of adjacent lumbar vertebrae in the procedure of *lumbar puncture* without damaging the spinal cord. A further consequence of the lag in growth rate of the spinal cord is related to the orientation of the spinal nerves. When the neural tube extends the whole length of the vertebral column a spinal nerve issuing from the lower part of the spinal cord passes out approximately horizontally through its own intervertebral foramen; as the spinal cord ascends relatively, however, the spinal nerves take an

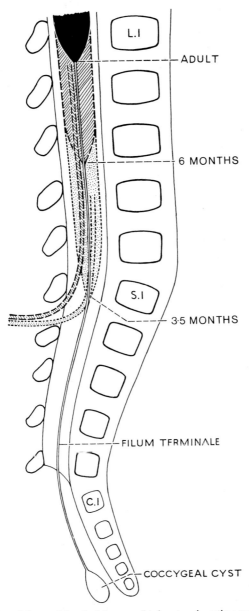

Fig. 99. The position of the caudal end of the neural tube at various time-periods. The vertebral canal is sectioned in the sagittal plane and viewed from the right side. The increasing inclination of the first sacral nerve is also demonstrated.

increasingly oblique course (Fig. 99) in order to issue from their corresponding intervertebral foramina, so producing elongated nerve roots inside
the subarachnoid space, which are collectively termed the *cauda equina.*

Development of brain vesicles

While the majority of the neural tube differentiates into the spinal cord, its
cephalic extremity undergoes differential dilatation to form the brain. At
first, three primary brain vesicles, the *prosencephalon, mesencephalon and
rhombencephalon* are differentiated. These parts of the developing brain are
also known as the fore-brain, mid-brain and hind-brain respectively (Fig.
100). The prosencephalon soon produces diverticula on either side at its
cephalic end to form the *telencephalic (cerebral) vesicles.* As a result, the
original fore-brain has now become divided into a telencephalon, composed
of telencephalic vesicles laterally and the telencephalon medium in the
mid-line which was originally the cephalic end of the prosencephalon, and
what remains of the prosencephalon, namely the *diencephalon* (Fig. 101).
Because the hind-brain kinks at a later stage in development it also becomes
divided into two parts—the part cephalic to the kink called the *metencephalon,* which will form the cerebellum, and a caudal part called the
myelencephalon which develops into the medulla oblongata.

The kinking of the hind-brain is just one event in the general bending of
the brain brought about by the fact that the neural tube continues to grow
from the caudal end of the embryo against a relatively fixed point (shown in
Fig. 102) where the bucco-pharyngeal membrane, the notochord and brain
meet. It will be remembered (p. 51) that it is around this point that flexion of
the head end of the embryo occurs. The development of the brain flexures
may also be caused by differential growth brought about by the development
of the telencephalon, and more extensive growth of the dorsal aspect of the
mesencephalon and rhombencephalon. The first such flexure to occur is at
the junction of brain and spinal cord and is called the cervical flexure. The
next occurs in the mid-brain and is therefore called the mesencephalic
flexure; this is formed at the same time as flexion of the head-end of the
embryo and may either cause or be brought about by the head flexion. The
final flexure occurs in the region of the hind-brain and is called the
hind-brain flexure or pontine flexure.

As an essential preliminary to describing details of the changes proceeding
in the development of the different parts of the brain it is necessary to
consider the overall changes seen by a gross examination of its lateral aspect.
The brain first consists of a simple tube with a cervical flexure at its junction
with the spinal cord and a mid-brain flexure. At its cephalic end there is a
small diverticulum on each side from the primitive fore-brain which is called
the *optic vesicle;* this will form the retina of the developing eye. On the lateral
aspect of the hind-brain neuromeres can be seen. The cervical and mid-brain
flexures become accentuated and the fore-brain can be seen more prominently

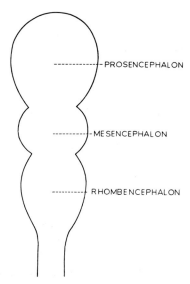

Fig. 100. The three primary brain vesicles.

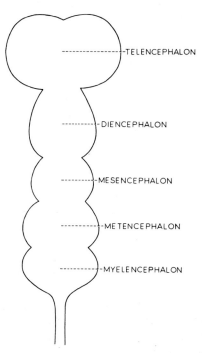

Fig. 101. Later stage in development of the brain vesicles in which the fore-brain and hind-brain show further differentiation.

as a differential dilatation. Already, at an early stage the optic vesicle has become invaginated to form the *optic cup*. Later, the pontine flexure appears and the hind-brain is now recognizably divided into a metencephalon and myelencephalon. The alar lamina of the metencephalon becomes very much enlarged and forms the cerebellum. At this stage also the telencephalic vesicles are beginning to develop. These vesicles form the cerebral

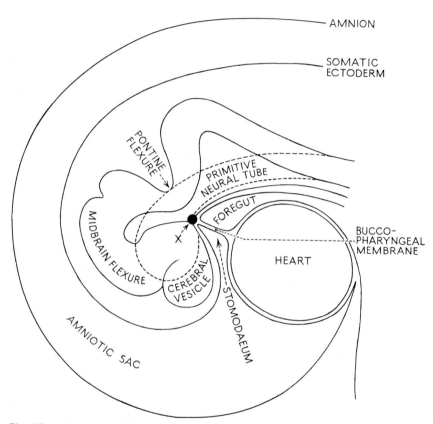

Fig. 102. A diagram of a median section through the embryo, viewed from the left side, to show the production of brain flexures. The neural tube when first a straight tube is indicated in dotted outline. X is the relatively fixed point against which growth of the neural tube produces the flexures, and around which flexion of the embryonic head occurs.

hemispheres and grow principally in an anterior, superior and posterior direction, so that they overlap the diencephalon. The diencephalon becomes differentiated and small diverticula occur from its floor and roof to form the posterior lobe of the pituitary gland and the pineal gland, respectively. The pineal evagination marks the caudal limit of the diencephalon. A small diverticulum from the anterior end of the telencephalic vesicle develops into the olfactory bulb and tract.

CLINICAL RELATIONSHIPS

If primitive streak cells persist and do not undergo necrosis together with general atrophy of the tail, a tumour may develop during fetal life. This tumour is termed a sacro-coccygeal teratoma and may grow to a large size, in which case it may present an obstruction to normal birth. It is attached to the lower end of the vertebral column and may be as big as the head of the newborn child. The tumour consists of a disorganized collection of tissues which develop from all germ layers; cartilage, nervous tissue, hair, teeth, thyroid gland tissue, a piece of pancreas, for example, may be found admixed in the tumour in disorderly fashion. The defect is due to persistence of primitive streak cells which then undergo unregulated activity owing to absence of normal organizer influence. Suggestions that such tumours represent an abortive effort to form a twin are unacceptable. A similar lack of normal regulated organizer influence is probably responsible for the development of an ovarian teratoma, and probably the not uncommon dermoid cyst of the ovary is to be included in this category. Such tumours are also known to occur in the testes, anterior mediastinum, retroperitoneal or mesenteric connective tissue, and in the presacral region. Some of these tumours are cystic and benign, whilst others are solid or polycystic and malignant.

One extraordinary condition which sometimes accompanies spina bifida is diastematomyelia, in which the spinal cord is divided into two parts, each part having its own central canal. This condition is also known to accompany the type of diplospondyly in which the two halves of the vertebral body are divided by a sagittal fissure.

References

Barson, A. J. (1970). The vertebral level of termination of the spinal cord during normal and abnormal development. *J. Anat.* **106,** 489-498.

Bergquist, H. and Källén, B. (1954). Notes on the early histogenesis and morphogenesis of the central nervous system in vertebrates. *J. comp. Neurol.* **100,** 627-659.

Neal, H. V. (1918). Neuromeres and metameres. *J. Morph.* **31,** 293-315.

Streeter, G. L. (1919). Factors involved in the formation of the filum terminale. *Am. J. Anat.* **25,** 1-11.

19

The Development of the Brain

Development of the hind-brain

When the hind-brain kinks, a change in cross-sectional appearance of the neural tube must occur. The lateral walls of the tube become separated and the roof plate is stretched and very much thinned, as shown in Fig. 103; consequently the columns of neuroblasts also become splayed out. The most lateral column in the greater part of the brain stem is the general somatic afferent and is concerned with the reception of sensory impulses from the skin of the head; the cranial nerve nucleus in this column is the sensory nucleus of the trigeminal which can therefore be classed as a general somatic afferent nucleus. The general somatic efferent column of neuroblasts is most medially situated and is associated with the propagation of impulses to musculature derived from somites, just as in the spinal cord; in the mid-brain and hind-brain the cranial nerve nuclei concerned are the IIIrd, IVth, VIth and XIIth. The first three of these cranial nerves innervate the orbital muscles which develop from the myotomes of somites lying in front of the otic capsule, a structure which forms the internal ear. The XIIth cranial or hypoglossal nerve in the embryo innervates somites lying in the occipital region. The myotomes of these somites later migrate forwards, producing a prominent epipericardial ridge above the developing heart and pericardium by so doing, and form the intrinsic and extrinsic musculature of the tongue; the hypoglossal grows forwards in the ridge to supply them. There are no discrete columns of neuroblasts in the mid-brain and hind-brain concerned with the propagation or reception of sympathetic nervous system impulses. The general splanchnic afferent and efferent columns of neuroblasts in the brain stem associated with the autonomic nervous system are related to the parasympathetic nervous system. The general splanchnic efferent column of neuroblasts is responsible for the propagation of impulses in the para-sympathetic components of certain cranial nerves, the IIIrd (Edinger-Westphal nucleus), VIIth and IXth (Salivatory nucleus) and Xth (Dorsal motor nucleus), while the general splanchnic afferent column of neuroblasts receives sensory impulses travelling in the parasympathetic components of the IXth and Xth cranial nerves.

In the head and neck there are nerves associated with the pharyngeal arches. Each of the pharyngeal arches forms well-defined structures and each arch has its own nerve of supply. The first pharyngeal arch is innervated by the Vth cranial nerve, the second by the VIIth, the third by the IXth and the fourth and sixth by the Xth. These cranial nerves have a special column of neuroblasts in the brain stem lying in between the general somatic and splanchnic afferent columns in the alar lamina and the general somatic and splanchnic efferent columns of neuroblasts in the basal lamina, the *special splanchnic afferent and efferent columns,* respectively. The Vth, VIIth, IXth and Xth cranial nerves have parts of their nuclei which are associated with the special splanchnic (or visceral) efferent column (this column is sometimes

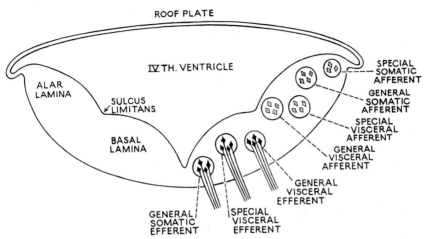

ROOF PLATE

IVTH. VENTRICLE

ALAR LAMINA

SULCUS LIMITANS

BASAL LAMINA

GENERAL SOMATIC EFFERENT

SPECIAL VISCERAL EFFERENT

GENERAL VISCERAL EFFERENT

GENERAL VISCERAL AFFERENT

SPECIAL VISCERAL AFFERENT

GENERAL SOMATIC AFFERENT

SPECIAL SOMATIC AFFERENT

Fig. 103. Diagrammatic transverse section through the hind-brain after formation of the pontine flexure showing the alar and basal laminae with their columns of neuroblasts.

termed the special somatic efferent column (see Brodal, 1969)). The nuclei of the IXth and Xth cranial nerves in this column are closely associated together as a single nucleus called the *nucleus ambiguus.* Sensory impulses which are derived from pharyngeal arch structures are received by the special visceral afferent column; thus the chorda tympani branch of the VIIth cranial nerve conveys the sensation of taste from the anterior two-thirds of the tongue and its fibres end in a nucleus which is combined with the other two cranial nerve nuclei to be found in this column, namely parts of the IXth and Xth, to form the *nucleus of the tractus solitarius.* A knowledge of this scheme of embryonic arrangement of neuroblasts in the primitive brain helps considerably the appreciation of the cranial nerves and their nuclei in the adult. The nucleus of VIII is described as special somatic afferent, and lies lateral to the general somatic afferent column.

The most lateral aspect of the alar lamina in the hind-brain is a very specialized region called the *rhombic lip;* this has the capacity of active mitosis and provides large numbers of neuroblasts which migrate cephalically into the ventral aspect of the hind-brain where they form the pontine nuclei and also slightly caudal to form the olivary nuclear complex. This streaming of neuroblasts from the rhombic lip in the hind-brain is so prominent a feature that it is called the corpus pontobulbare. Harkmark (1954) has found it possible to remove the rhombic lip in chick embryos; the resulting grown chicks lack an inferior olive and pontine nuclei, so providing evidence that the rhombic lip is concerned with the production of these nuclei.

While differentiation is proceeding in the myelencephalon, a proliferation of tissue occurs in each alar lamina of the metencephalon. These proliferations which are at first intraventricular—i.e. into the cavity of the neural tube at this point, which will form the fourth ventricle—meet and fuse to form the cerebellum. The lateral contributions form the hemispheres and their point of fusion the vermis, of the cerebellum; later it becomes extraventricular and can be seen on the external aspect of the brain.

Development of the mid-brain

The mesencephalon develops just in front of the hind-brain and although it lies at the site of a bend, the mesencephalic flexure, its cavity does not become kinked like that of the hind-brain because the flexure is not so acute. In other words, its cavity remains relatively unchanged as the aqueduct although at first it has a prominent sulcus limitans dividing the alar lamina dorsally from the basal lamina ventrally. The roof of the mid-brain first thickens on each side of the mid-line to form two longitudinal elevations. These undergo transverse constriction to form four bodies, the corpora quadrigemina, which are reflex centres for sight and hearing. At the same time, there is a congregation of neuroblasts in the basal lamina to form two nuclei, the red nucleus and the substantia nigra. The latter is so called because it really is black, as can be seen even in the unstained brain, due to the fact that its component cells contain melanin granules. The mid-brain can be divided into two parts, the dorsal aspect or the tectum, which is merely another name for the roof of this part of the brain, and a ventral portion derived from the basal lamina which is called the tegmentum. On the ventral aspect of this, certain nerve tracts later become applied one after another (Fig. 104); these tracts place various parts of the brain in communication one with another. The development of the mesencephalon is, therefore, dependent on the differentiation of other parts of the brain and when the tracts develop and pass up to or down from different levels of the central nervous system, they become applied on to the ventral aspect of the mid-brain. The first nerve tract which becomes associated with the tegmentum in this way is the medial longitudinal fasciculus, an association tract connecting certain cranial nerve nuclei. The next nerve tracts to become applied constitute the lemnisci, composed of nerve fibres passing up to the thalamus from the gracile and cuneate nuclei as the medial lemnisci, or travelling in the lateral lemnisci from the cochlear nuclei to the medial geniculate bodies and decussating fibres from the cerebellum to the red nuclei. Finally, since the cerebral cortex is late to develop, corticopontine and corticospinal (pyramidal) fibres pass down on the ventral aspect of the substantia nigra as the crus cerebri which, together with the tegmentum, forms the cerebral peduncle on each side.

Development of the fore-brain

The diencephalon is that part of the fore-brain remaining in the midline after the telencephalic vesicles grow out from the fore-brain, overlap the

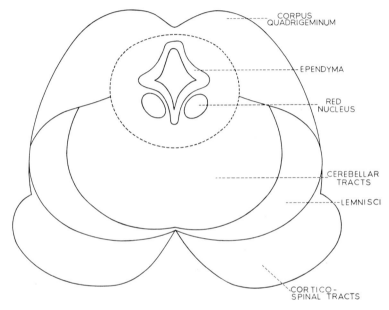

Fig. 104. A diagram showing the development of the mesencephalon in cross-section. The dotted outline represents the mid-brain in early development.

diencephalon and compress it (Fig. 105). The cavity of the diencephalon becomes the third ventricle of the adult brain; its lateral wall develops three bulges, with sulci in between, which are, from above downwards, the epithalamus, the thalamus and the hypothalamus. The thalamus is separated from the epithalamus by the epithalamic sulcus and from the hypothalamus by the hypothalamic sulcus. The diencephalon is in communication with each telencephalic vesicle by a foramen which is very large at first, and is called the interventricular foramen. At the cephalic extremity of the diencephalon is the telencephalon medium whose anterior wall forms a thickened plate, the lamina terminalis, which lies at the most anterior extremity of the adult brain. The epithalamus is a well-developed nuclear mass in the lateral wall of the diencephalon in the early part of development but it soon diminishes relatively in size because later (Dekaban, 1954) the thalamus differentiates and grows much more rapidly and becomes the largest nuclear mass in the lateral wall of the third ventricle.

The thalamus later contacts its fellow across the midline and establishes a connection with it called the adhesio interthalamica (interthalamic connexus), which does not contain, however, any nerve fibres. The thalamus is a

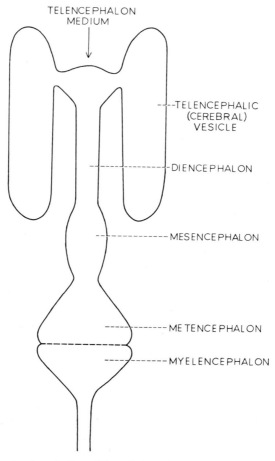

Fig. 105. Diagram to show further differentiation of the brain vesicles to produce the telencephalic vesicles.

collection of nerve cells which later become divided into separate nuclei connected with the spinal cord and other parts of the central nervous system. Its caudal nuclei form the geniculate bodies. The hypothalamus also lags behind to a certain extent in development but not as much as the epithalamus; in it develop nuclei which are concerned with involuntary actions and movements, such as sleep. The hypothalamus has been called the head ganglion of the sympathetic nervous system. From the floor of the diencephalon, a small diverticulum develops called the *infundibulum,* which will form the stalk and posterior lobe of the pituitary gland. The anterior lobe of the pituitary gland is formed from *Rathke's pouch,* which develops as a diverticulum upwards from the stomodaeum. At one point in development, the diencephalon and the ectoderm of the stomodaeum are in very close relationship as shown in Fig. 102, so that it is very easy for any diverticulum from the stomodaeum to come in contact with the infundibulum. A *craniopharyngeal canal* is present frequently in the human newborn and although it pursues the same general course as the pathway of Rathke's pouch, no direct relationship exists between the two, since the canal is formed secondarily during ossification of the skull base (Arey, 1950). Yet accessory pituitary tissue may be found in the pharyngeal end of the canal (Boyd, 1956).

Because the posterior lobe of the pituitary gland develops as a downgrowth from the hypothalamus, it is composed of modified neuroglial cells called pituicytes and remains in communication with the hypothalamic nuclei by means of certain nerve tracts, such as the supraoptico-hypophysial tract. Since the anterior lobe of the pituitary gland develops from somatic ectoderm, not from the central nervous system, there are no nerve fibres passing into it from the hypothalamus in adult life. Yet the pars anterior is under the influence of the hypothalamus by means of the hypophysial portal system of blood vessels. The original anterior wall of Rathke's pouch proliferates very considerably to form the pars anterior. The posterior wall, however, does not proliferate so markedly and forms the pars intermedia. These two parts of the gland are separated by the original cavity of Rathke's pouch which forms the narrow slit (intraglandular cleft) in the substance of the pituitary.

A knowledge of the structure of the roof of the reptilian fore-brain helps understanding of the development of the roof of the diencephalon (Warren, 1917). Most anteriorly, there is a stalked glandular structure called the *paraphysis* (Fig. 106); this disappears completely in human development and probably does not represent the sub-fornical organ of mammals (Legait and Legait, 1957), although a few cells may remain behind in the upper part of the lamina terminalis. Most so-called "paraphyseal cystic tumours" do not have a paraphyseal origin but develop from detached undegenerated embryonic ependymal vesicular recesses (Kappers, 1955). Immediately behind this is an invagination called the *velum transversum* which is also seen as an invagination of the roof of the human diencephalon to form the choroid plexus. Behind this is the *dorsal sac* which merely forms the roof of the third ventricle. The most caudal structure in the roof of the reptilian diencephalon is a complex of structures; the *parapineal,* in front of which is a commissure, called the habenular commissure, and behind which is the *pineal gland,* posterior to which is the posterior commissure. The two commissures persist in man; the parapineal, which probably represents the parietal eye in reptiles, disappears and is not present even in the human embryo but the pineal gland persists as such in adult man. The functions of the pineal have been reviewed by Altschule (1975).

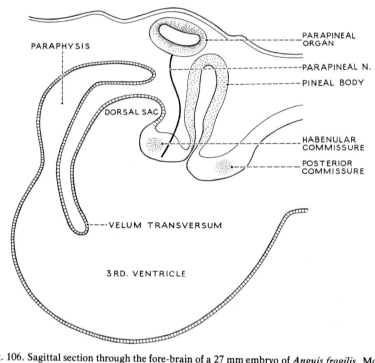

Fig. 106. Sagittal section through the fore-brain of a 27 mm embryo of *Anguis fragilis.* Modified from Tilney and Warren (1919).

The telencephalon

The telencephalic or cerebral vesicles form the cerebral hemispheres. They appear as diverticula from the prosencephalon and overlap the lateral aspect of the diencephalon but remain in communication with it by means of a wide interventricular foramen. A coronal section through this foramen has the appearance shown in Figs 107 and 108. The wall of the inferior aspect of the vesicle first thickens to form a structure called the *corpus striatum;* the remainder of the cerebral vesicle can therefore be called the *supra-striatal portion,* or *pallium.* The attachment of the telencephalon to the upper part of the diencephalon next proliferates and invaginates into the cavity of the cerebral vesicle to form the choroid plexus, the site of invagination being the choroid fissure; the cavity of the cerebral vesicle becomes the lateral ventricle. The pallium just above the choroid fissure then begins to thicken and forms the *hippocampus;* the part of the pallium just lateral to the corpus striatum forms the *piriform cortex,* including the *uncus,* the olfactory sensory area of the cerebral cortex. When this happens, the remainder of the pallium is now called the *neo-pallium.* The hippocampus differentiates first because it is the most primitive part of the pallium.

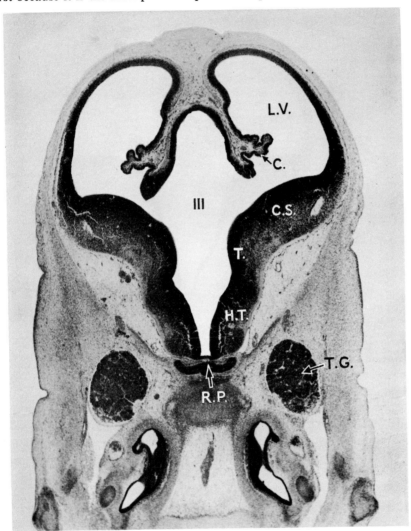

Fig. 107. The diencephalon (III) and telencephalic vesicles (L.V.) of an 11·2 mm human embryo shown in transverse section at the level of the interventricular foramen. The choroid plexus (C.) is clearly shown, and in the floor of the lateral ventricle (which is developing from the cavity of the telencephalon), the corpus striatum (C.S.). Eminences in the lateral wall of the diencephalon are forming the thalamus (T.) and hypothalamus (H.T.). Rathke's pouch (R.P.) is seen lying ventral to the diencephalon, and the trigeminal ganglion (T.G.) is visible on each side. (× 24).

The neo-pallium later thickens considerably and neuroblasts differentiate within it. From these neuroblasts nerve fibres pass down to lower levels as the corticospinal tract. This and other corticofugal and corticopetal tracts grow through the corpus striatum and divide it into two parts: a lateral part or *lentiform nucleus* and a medial *caudate nucleus* (see Hewitt, 1961). Where the tracts pass through the corpus striatum they are called the *internal*

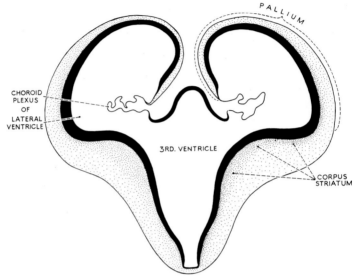

Fig. 108. A diagram of a coronal section through the diencephalon and telencephalon at the level of the interventricular foramen.

capsule (Fig. 109). The head of the caudate nucleus shows further development by the successive appearance of three striatal elevations (Hewitt, 1958). Because of the great development of the neo-pallium the hippocampus lags behind in development and remains as the hippocampal formation in adult life. Finally, nerve fibres connect the two cerebral hemispheres to form the various commissures. The growth of the neo-pallium in the wall of the cerebral vesicle also constricts its cavity so that it comes to take the shape of the adult lateral ventricle.

The growth of the cerebral vesicle in this process occurs only in an anterior, superior and posterior direction (Fig. 110). There is a region in the middle of the cerebral hemisphere which does not appear to grow at all rapidly; it lags behind in development and comes to be overlapped by the other portions of the cerebral hemisphere. The parts of the cerebral hemisphere which overlap it are called the *opercula* and the portion of the cerebral cortex which therefore becomes sunk below the surface of the brain is called the insula. This manner of growth of the cerebral hemisphere is

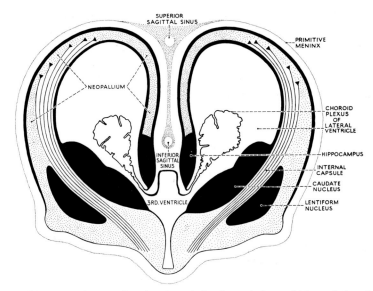

Fig. 109. Diagrammatic coronal section through the diencephalon and telencephalon at a stage when neuroblasts in the neopallium have produced nerve fibres which pass down to lower levels as the corticospinal tract and divide the corpus striatum into two parts as the internal capsule.

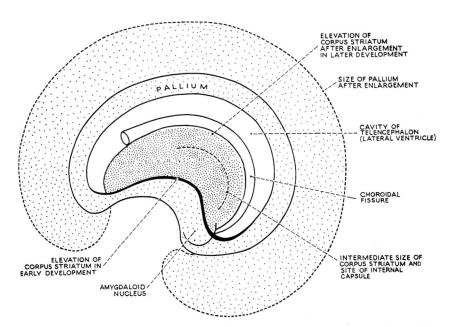

Fig. 110. A diagram to show how the growth of the corpus striatum changes the shape of the lateral ventricle during development of the telencephalic vesicle to ensure formation of the inferior horn of the lateral ventricle.

probably related to the direction of growth of the corpus striatum; a sagittal section (Fig. 110) through the cerebral hemisphere shows that the corpus striatum bulges upwards and backwards; as a result the shape of the lateral ventricle is changed and the posterior aspect of it becomes curved (Fig. 111), so forming the inferior horn of the lateral ventricle in the temporal lobe of the brain which in this way comes into existence: The corpus striatum comes

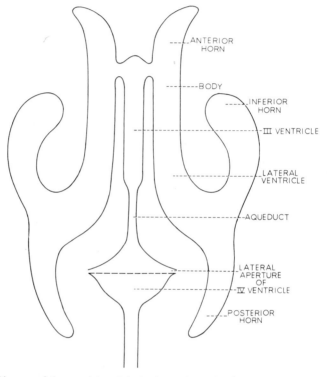

Fig. 111. Diagram of the ventricles of the brain produced from the cerebral vesicles.

to lie in the roof of the inferior horn of the lateral ventricle. Similarly, the choroid fissure also becomes curved in conformity with the curve of the ventricle itself. The growth of the corpus striatum, together with an "invagination" of the diencephalon into the telencephalon, constricts the interventricular foramen and changes its shape from circular to oval (Sharp, 1959).

It remains to mention the histogenesis of the wall of the cerebral hemisphere. In the primitive neural tube the neuroblasts are congregated in the mantle zone of the tube. Later in the development of the human cerebrum, these neuroblasts migrate to the periphery of the tube and so form the grey matter which lies on the external aspect of the cerebrum. The grey matter therefore comes to occupy the marginal zone of the neural tube and the nerve fibres to which its cells give origin pass centripetally instead of centrifugally as in the spinal cord. A similar process occurs in the cerebellum.

The formation of the insula and opercula also ensures the development of the lateral sulcus; the forces which are primarily responsible for the development of other sulci are resident in the cortex and the folding of the cerebral cortex is *not* due to a disproportion between (a) the rate of increase in capacity of the cranial cavity and the mass of the cerebrum and (b) the rate of increase of cortical surface relative to the underlying structures of the telencephalon and diencephalon (Barron, 1950).

CLINICAL RELATIONSHIPS

A major part of the brain, usually the cerebral hemispheres at least, may fail to develop, a condition termed *anencephaly,* occurring 1:800-1600 births. There may also be an accentuation of the degenerative processes which normally occur to a certain extent in development (p. 184). The membranous neurocranium also shows faulty development in this disorder, so that the skull vault is lacking *(acrania)*. Various regions of the brain may show faulty development. If the motor cortex fails to develop, a spastic paralysis is evident in the newborn child; minor defects of development may also occur. Thus lack of development of association fibres which subserve the association between sounds and other sensory impressions will result in congenital word-deafness (congenital auditory imperception). Although hearing is normal, spoken language is not understood and speech suffers seriously. Similarly, developmental alexia may occur, in which there is a defect in learning to read. If extensive lack of development of the cerebral cortex occurs, the child is born a congenital idiot.

The brain may be larger (megaloencephaly) or smaller (micrencephaly) than normal. These conditions are associated with a large (macrocephaly) or small (microcephaly) cranium. Estimation of cranial capacity gives an estimate of brain volume, and it is extremely variable in the adult, from 1000 to 1800 cm^3 (mean 1400 cm^3). The vermis of the cerebellum may fail to develop, and the corpus callosum may be absent either in whole or in part. One cerebellar hemisphere may fail to develop.

In *hydrocephalus* there is an excessive enlargement of the cerebral ventricles accompanied by an increase in volume of cerebrospinal fluid. The resultant generalized increase in C.S.F. pressure compresses the brain against the relatively unexpandable skull with resultant brain damage. If present for some time before birth the skull is enlarged, with separation of sutures and an enlarged anterior fontanelle. The condition is often due to congenital narrowing, or stenosis, of the cerebral aqueduct by overgrowth of glial tissue around it. Maldevelopment of the interventricular foramina or defective absorption of C.S.F. may occur with the same result. In the latter, there is increased cerebral venous pressure, and decreased cerebral blood flow; the resulting ischaemia causes necrosis of the white matter and therefore "thinning" of the cerebral cortex.

References

Altschule, M. D. (1975). "Frontiers of Pineal Physiology" M.I.T. Press, London.

Arey, L. B. (1950). The craniopharyngeal canal reviewed and reinterpreted. *Anat. Rec.* **106**, 1-16.

Barron, D. H. (1950). An experimental analysis of some factors involved in the development of the fissure pattern of the cerebral cortex. *J. exp. Zool.* **113**, 553-582.

Boyd, J. D. (1956). Observations on the human pharyngeal hypophysis. *J. Endocr.* **14**, 66-77.

Brodal, A. (1969). "Neurological Anatomy in Relation to Clinical Medicine" 2nd. edn. Oxford University Press.

Dekaban, A. (1954). Human thalamus. An anatomical, developmental and pathological study. II. Development of the human thalamic nuclei. *J. comp. Neurol.* **100**, 63-98.

Harkmark, W. (1954). Cell migrations from the rhombic lip to the inferior olive, the nucleus raphe and the pons. A morphological and experimental investigation on chick embryos. *J. comp. Neurol.* **102**, 425-510.

Hewitt, W. (1958). The development of the human caudate and amygdaloid nuclei. *J. Anat.* **92**, 377-382.

Hewitt, W. (1961). The development of the human internal capsule and lentiform nucleus. *J. Anat.* **95**, 191-199.

Kappers, J. A. (1955). The development of the paraphysis cerebri in man with comments on its relationship to the intercolumnar tubercle and its significance for the origin of cystic tumours in the third ventricle. *J. comp. Neurol.* **102**, 425-510.

Legait, H. and Legait, E. (1957). Paraphyse et organe sub-fornical chez les oiseaux. *C.r.seanc. Soc. Biol.* **151**, 365-367.

Sharp, J. A. (1959). Developmental changes in the interventricular foramen. *J. Anat.* **93**, 23-29.

Tilney, F. and Warren, L. F. (1919). The morphology and evolutional significance of the pineal body. *The American Anatomical Memoirs* **9**, 1-256.

Warren, J. (1917). The development of the paraphysis and pineal region in mammalia. *J. comp. Neurol.* **28**, 75-136.

20

The Relation of the Cranial Nerves to the Development of the Pharyngeal Arches

Pharyngeal arch derivatives

Some of the cranial nerves supply the pharyngeal arches and since certain structures develop from these arches, in adult life they are innervated by the cranial nerves supplying the arches.

It has already been mentioned (p. 116) that different areas of the face are derived from the mandibular and maxillary processes of the first pharyngeal arch and also from the frontonasal process. Each of these processes has its own nerve supply, a division of the trigeminal nerve. Areas of the adult face are innervated by sensory twigs from each of the three divisions of the Vth cranial nerve (Fig. 112). The first and second pharyngeal arches contain cartilages, the cartilage of the first arch being called *Meckel's cartilage*. The mesoderm of the mandibular process condenses around Meckel's cartilage and undergoes intramembranous ossification to form the mandible. Meckel's cartilage itself takes no part in the formation of the mandible and disappears, except for certain structures which persist into adult life. The dorsal end of the cartilage remains as one of the ossicles in the middle ear cavity—the malleus; its sheath also persists as the sphenomandibular ligament and the anterior ligament of of the malleus. The tensor tympani muscle is attached to the malleus and since it develops from the first pharyngeal arch it is innervated by the mandibular nerve. Other muscles also develop from this arch, notably the muscles of mastication and the anterior belly of the digastric muscle; they are also therefore supplied by the mandibular nerve. Since the connective tissue and mucous membrane of the anterior two-thirds of the tongue also develops from the mandibular arch, it is innervated for every sensation except taste by the lingual nerve, which is a branch of the mandibular nerve.

The sensation of taste in the anterior two-thirds of the tongue is mediated by the chorda tympani nerve and this is a branch of the facial nerve, which is the nerve of the second pharyngeal arch. Such an innervation is understandable because the chorda tympani is the *pretrematic* (i.e. passing anterior to the first pharyngeal groove and pouch) *branch* of the facial nerve supplying the first arch, the facial nerve itself being the post-trematic nerve to the second arch. The post-trematic nerve to the first arch is the mandibular nerve itself. The maxillary process of the mandibular arch has as its nerve of supply the maxillary nerve (second division of the trigeminal). This process also has a cartilage which is called the *pterygoquadrate* (*palatoquadrate*) *bar* which disappears entirely except for the fact that it forms the incus, another of the ossicles of the middle ear.

The second pharyngeal arch cartilage is called *Reichert's cartilage* and this forms a variety of structures. At its dorsal end it develops into the stapes, the third of the middle ear ossicles. It also forms the styloid process of the skull, the lesser horn of the hyoid bone and the upper part of the body of the hyoid.

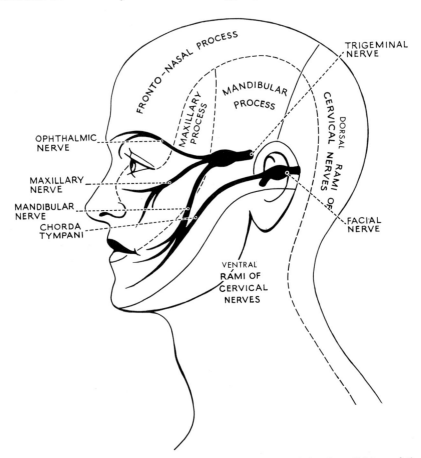

Fig. 112. The areas of the face innervated by sensory branches of the three divisions of the trigeminal nerve. The chorda tympani joins on to the lingual branch of the mandibular division of the trigeminal nerve to be distributed to the taste buds of the anterior two-thirds of the tongue and therefore supply special sensation there.

Its sheath develops into the stylohyoid ligament. The muscle which is attached to the stapes, namely the stapedius muscle, the muscles of facial expression, the posterior belly of the digastric muscle and the stylo-hyoid muscle, are all derived from the second arch mesoderm and are therefore supplied by the facial nerve. The third pharyngeal arch is innervated by the glossopharyngeal nerve and its cartilage forms the lower part of the body and the greater horn of the hyoid bone. There is only one muscle which properly develops from this arch, namely the stylopharyngeus muscle, which is therefore supplied by the glossopharyngeal nerve. Since the connective tissue and mucous membrane of the posterior third of the tongue are derived from the third arch the sensory supply of this part of the tongue for ordinary sensation and taste is mediated by the glossopharyngeal nerve.

The fourth pharyngeal arch is innervated by the superior laryngeal branch of the vagus. The cricothyroid muscle and the constrictors of the pharynx also develop from this arch and are therefore innervated by this particular nerve. Although the cricothyroid muscle is innervated by the external laryngeal nerve, which is a branch of the superior laryngeal nerve, the fibres of the latter supplying the constrictors of the pharynx are probably derived from the cranial root of the accessory nerve, distributed through the superior laryngeal. The thyroid cartilage of the larynx also develops from this region. The posterior part of the tongue, in the region of the vallecula epiglottica, is derived from the fourth arch and its sensory innervation is therefore provided by the internal laryngeal nerve. The fifth pharyngeal arch is a transitory structure and disappears almost as soon as it is formed. The sixth pharyngeal arch, however, does persist and its nerve of supply is the recurrent laryngeal branch of the vagus. It is not surprising, therefore, that the intrinsic musculature of the larynx, except the cricothyroid muscle, and the cricoid and arytenoid cartilages of the larynx, also develop from this arch.

In certain animals, particularly the carnivores and ungulates, the hyoid bone is a complicated structure forming the so-called hyoid apparatus (Fig. 113), which consists of several independent elements. Of these separate elements the tympanohyal and the stylohyal develop into the styloid process. The ceratohyal forms the lesser horn of the hyoid bone and also develops into the upper part of the body of the hyoid. The epihyal does not form a bone in the human being but becomes incorporated in the stylohyoid ligament. The thyrohyal which develops from the third arch, differentiates into the greater horn and lower part of the body of the hyoid bone.

The position of the embryonic ectodermal pharyngeal clefts can be represented in the adult as shown in Fig. 114.

CLINICAL RELATIONSHIPS

A small anomalous nodule of bone is occasionally found in the stylohyoid ligament. This is often described as a heteropic or pathological ossification when it occurs, but this is unlikely, since it is more probably the result of persistence of the epihyal and therefore of a more primitive embryonic condition.

The first and second pharyngeal arches grow more rapidly than the third or

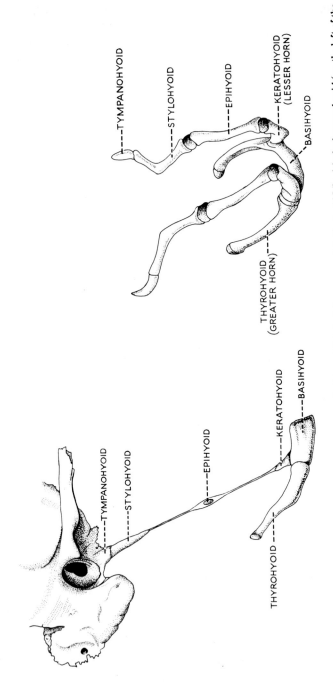

Fig. 113. A diagram comparing the hyoid apparatus of a dog (modified from Nickel, Schummer and Seiferle, 1954) with the human hyoid (on the left of the figure).

fourth. In consequence the second arch grows backwards externally, over the surface of the more caudal arches. The second, third and fourth clefts, therefore, become depressed from the surface as an ectodermally lined sinus—the *cervical sinus,* which may persist to open on the surface of the neck just anterior to the sternal head of origin of the sternocleidomastoid muscle (Fig. 114). Normally, however, it completely disappears, and the

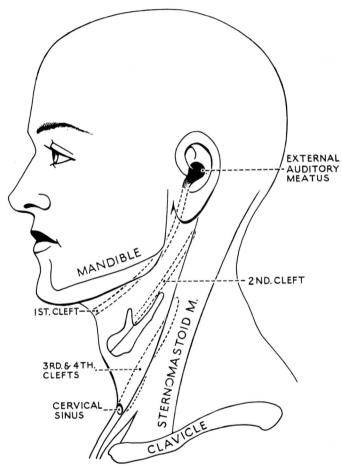

Fig. 114. The relative position of the pharyngeal ectodermal clefts in the adult. The cervical sinus is shown passing deep to the sternocleidomastoid (sternomastoid) muscle, and the external acoustic (auditory) meatus is seen developing from the dorsal extremity of the first pharyngeal cleft.

third and fourth pharyngeal clefts are obliterated. These clefts, however, persist independently as vesicles for a while and become completely closed off from the surface. Such *cervical vesicles* may also arise from the second cleft. Abnormally these vesicles persist into adult life as *cervical (branchial) cysts.*

Since the ectoderm in the depths of the third and fourth clefts normally thickens to form placodes which contribute sensory nerve cells to the ganglia of the glossopharyngeal and vagus nerves, it may be presumed that cervical cysts, when they occur, are closely related to the IXth and Xth nerves. As might be expected, their position is fairly constant, lying deep to the sternocleidomastoid, in contact with the carotid sheath at the level of the hyoid bone. Occasionally a branchial cyst may be attached to the pharynx internally by a pedicle which passes in between the external and internal carotid arteries, or to the skin anterior to the sternocleidomastoid externally by a similar pedicle. The external skin attachment may be regarded as an abortive cervical sinus. In similar fashion an internal cervical sinus, representing the internal pedicle of a cervical cyst, occurs rarely. It also passes upwards between internal and external carotid arteries and opens into the pharynx at the tonsillar fossa. Occasionally a branchial (pharyngo-cutaneous) fistula may occur communicating internally with the pharynx, and opening externally on the neck anterior to sternocleidomastoid. This disorder must clearly depend on the breakdown of the closing membrane corresponding to the pharyngeal cleft in question.

Reference

Nickel, R., Schummer, A. and Seiferle, E. (1954). "Lehrbuch der Anatomie der Haustiere" Band 1. Paul Parey, Berlin and Hamburg.

21

The Pharynx and the Special Senses

Development of the eye

The first, second and eighth cranial nerves are the nerves of the special senses and develop in association with the structures they supply. Thus, the development of the optic nerve cannot be understood until the development of the eye itself is described (for details see Mann, 1949).

The first sign of the developing eye is a diverticulum of the fore-brain called the *optic vesicle*. This then becomes invaginated from its anterior and inferior aspect to form the *optic cup*. As a result of this the original one-layered optic vesicle now becomes a two-layered optic cup (Fig. 115), which then produces organizers to act on the overlying ectoderm and cause the induction of the lens. (Amprino (1951) has, however, found no indication of such an inductive activity on periocular organs such as the eyelids, lacrimal glands and nasolacrimal duct.) This first appears as a thickening of the ectoderm, the *lens placode*, which then sinks below the surface to form a pit, the *fovea lentis;* the fovea rounds off to form a cyst, the *lens vesicle,* which develops into the lens of the eye. The invaginating process affects not only the optic vesicle but also its connection with the brain, the *optic stalk.* When the optic stalk becomes invaginated a small artery, which is a branch of the ophthalmic artery, passes along it to reach the lens and vascularize it (Fig. 116); this is the *hyaloid artery,* and the fissure in the optic stalk in which it lies is therefore called the hyaloid fissure which later closes inferiorly so enclosing the artery. The optic cup is destined to form only the retina of the eye. In the adult retina there are two layers, an outer pigmented layer and an inner nervous layer (Fig. 115). The pigmented layer is formed from the outer layer of the optic cup and the nervous layer from the inner layer. The two layers are separated by a space, the intraretinal space, which is the cavity of the original optic vesicle. It will be remembered that the layers of the neural tube, from which, of course, the optic vesicle develops are, from within outwards, the ependymal zone, the mantle zone and the marginal zone. When the vesicle becomes invaginated to form the optic cup, the inner (nervous) layer of the cup therefore has the ependymal zone outermost and it is this layer which differentiates into the rods and cones of the retina; the mantle zone develops into the bipolar cells and the marginal zone into the ganglionic layer. The apparently paradoxical disposition of the light-sensitive cells in the outermost layer of the retina is therefore explained on embryological grounds.

The lens vesicle comes to sink into the cavity of the optic cup and originally has a wide open cavity. The cells in the posterior wall of the lens vesicle then lengthen considerably (Fig. 117), so forming the lens fibres of the adult lens and thereby obliterate the cavity of the vesicle. The cells of the anterior wall of the lens vesicle do not change appreciably, however, and form the anterior epithelial layer of the lens. Mesoderm migrates into the space between the overlying somatic ectoderm and the lens as the corneal mesoderm (Fig. 118), and this in turn forms two layers—a thick layer underneath the ectoderm which develops into the cornea and a very thin layer of cells over the anterior aspect of the lens called the *pupillary membrane*. The cavity in the corneal mesoderm which separates the two layers forms the anterior chamber of the

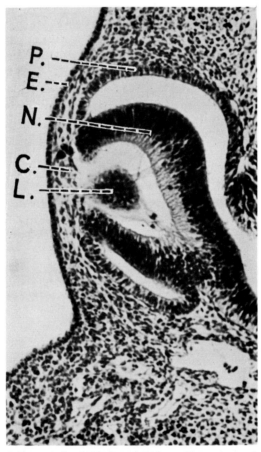

Fig. 115. The developing eye of a 7 mm human embryo. The optic cup has formed and the pigmented (P.) and nervous (N.) layers of the retina are clearly shown, separated by what was the cavity of the optic vesicle, which will form the intraretinal space. The lens (L.) has developed and mesoderm is visible on its deep aspect (probably the precursor of the hyaloid artery). The corneal mesoderm (C.) separates the lens from the somatic ectoderm (E.). The plane of section is to one side of the cavity of the lens vesicle. (× 115).

eye. The pupillary membrane normally disappears but if it persists it produces one form of congenital defect of the eye by remaining over the surface of the lens obscuring vision (for details of this and other abnormalities of the eye, see Mann, 1957).

The mesoderm also congregates around the optic cup. At one point it forms a small accumulation which indents the optic cup to form the ciliary body.

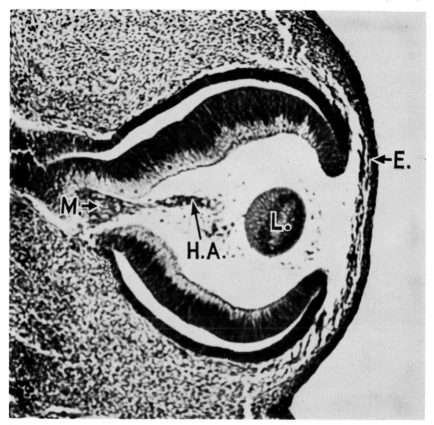

Fig. 116. Longitudinal section through the eye of a 13 mm human embryo. Mesoderm (M.) and the hyaloid artery (H.A.) are growing into the optic cup. The lens vesicle (L.) has sunk well below the surface ectoderm (E.) and its cavity has become obliterated (× 115).

When the ciliary body develops it divides the optic cup into two parts, a portion in front of it, the pars iridica retinae, which forms the iris and a portion behind it which develops into the pars optica retinae. In the adult iris there are two fundamental tissue components, muscular and pigmented, both developed from the iridal part of the optic cup. The iris musculature is therefore derived from ectoderm and this is one of the two sites in the body where this is known to occur; the other instance being the myoepithelial cells of the mammary and sweat glands.

Mesoderm surrounding the optic cup develops into the other two coats of the eye, namely the choroid and sclera. The mesoderm also infiltrates in between the iris and the lens and comes to occupy the cavity of the optic cup where it forms the vitreous body. The vitreous body surrounds the hyaloid artery, which atrophies when the lens is fully developed, so leaving a canal in the adult vitreous which is called the *hyaloid canal.* The proximal part of this artery up to the retina, however, persists as the central artery of the retina and gives off branches which ramify in the retina to vascularize it. Since the optic vesicle was originally invaginated from its anterior and inferior aspect,

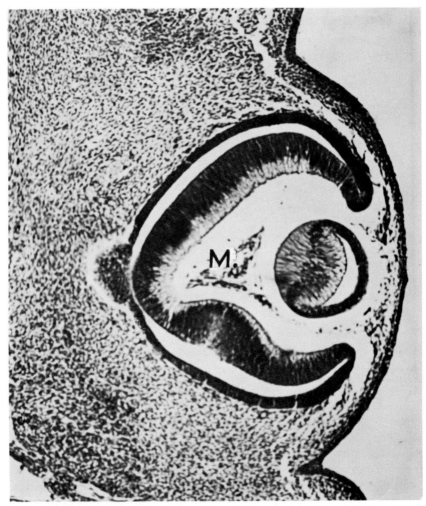

Fig. 117. Paramedian section through the eye of an 11·2 mm human embryo. Mesoderm (M.) is lying in the space between the lens vesicle and the nervous layer of the optic cup. The lens vesicle is showing lengthening of cells in its posterior wall to form lens fibres. (× 115).

the optic cup so formed must be closed off by growth at the margins of the hyaloid fissure. The eyelids develop as folds of ectoderm containing mesoderm superficial to the cornea; they fuse together and then separate before birth.

Development of the olfactory nerves

The olfactory nerves form in association with the development of the face and have already been mentioned. They develop from thickenings of the ectoderm called nasal placodes, which sink below the surface as the olfactory

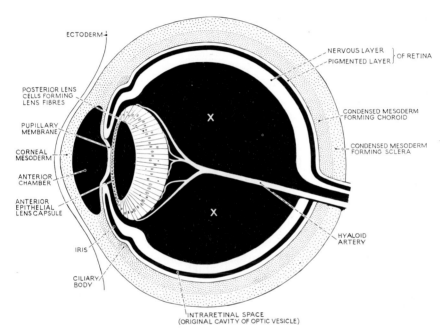

Fig 118 A diagram of a longitudinal section through the developing eye to show the vascularization of the embryonic lens by the hyaloid artery, which lies in the vitreous body (XX in figure). Mesoderm has surrounded the optic cup to develop into the choroid and sclera, and has infiltrated in between the iris and surface ectoderm where a cavity which has developed in it to form the anterior chamber separates the corneal mesoderm from the pupillary membrane. The mesoderm is also invaginating the retina just behind the iris to form the ciliary body.

pits. The ectoderm of the olfactory pits forms the mucous membrane lining the inside of the nasal cavity; the upper part of this mucous membrane differentiates into the olfactory epithelium in which the olfactory nerve fibres develop (see Planel, 1951). These nerve fibres enter the olfactory bulb, which, like the optic nerve and optic cup, is an outgrowth from the primitive brain and therefore a brain tract. The olfactory nerves are, therefore, rather interesting in that they are developed from somatic ectoderm.

Development of the ear. The pharynx and middle ear

The auditory (vestibulocochlear) nerves develop in association with the internal ear which becomes related to the middle ear cavity and since this is derived from the pharynx it is necessary to know something about the development of the pharynx itself. The appearance of the floor of the embryonic pharynx is shown in Fig. 41 and it may be noted that there are originally six pharyngeal arches, the fifth disappearing rather rapidly. The first arch does not quite cross the midline because of the presence of a small tubercle called the *tuberculum impar,* which is really part of the first arch. Similarly the third and fourth arches do not cross the midline because of an eminence in the floor of the pharynx, called the hypobranchial eminence. From the pharyngeal arches differentiate various structures already mentioned. The floor of the adult mouth and pharynx also develops from the floor of the embryonic pharynx.

The hypobranchial eminence develops into the epiglottis; this lies immediately anterior to the opening of the larynx which is formed from the laryngo-tracheal groove in between the sixth arches. From the tuberculum impar and the adjoining portions of the first arch, are derived the connective tissue and mucous membrane of the anterior two-thirds of the tongue. From the medial ends of the third arch, proliferations migrate forward over the second arches to meet the anterior two-thirds of the tongue and form the posterior one-third of the tongue. The thyroid gland also develops from the floor of the embryonic pharynx as a small diverticulum which grows downwards from a point immediately behind the tuberculum impar and in front of the second arch. It becomes bilobed and then attaches itself on to the common carotid arteries and as the heart "descends" it drags with it these arteries and also the thyroid gland, which therefore descends to its adult level. The original communication with the floor of the pharynx becomes attenuated and is called the *thyroglossal duct;* this is attached at its superior extremity to the point of original formation of the diverticulum which remains in the adult as the foramen caecum of the tongue. This foramen lies at the apex of a sulcus—the sulcus terminalis—which is a V-shaped groove at the site of junction of the anterior two-thirds with the posterior one-third of the tongue. The weight of human fetal thyroids in relation to the length, weight and age of the fetus is lower in smaller fetuses and increases until the embryo is about 3½ months old, when the ratio is similar to that found in the newborn and the adult; the relative weight becomes constant at the time when the ability to concentrate iodine appears (Sheppard, Andersen and Andersen, 1964a) and colloid is first found in fetal thyroid follicles (Sheppard, Andersen and Andersen, 1964b).

The lateral aspect of the pharynx has endodermal pouches and ectodermal clefts in between the arches (Fig. 41) from which other structures develop. The clefts are on the external aspect of the lateral wall of the pharynx while the pouches are on the internal aspect. The clefts and pouches are separated by the *closing membranes* which never break down in man to form gill slits. The first and second pharyngeal pouches are of particular importance, since they participate in the development of the ear. They enlarge and become confluent to form a diverticulum from the dorso-lateral aspect of the pharynx which is called the *tubo-tympanic recess (diverticulum)*. As its name suggests, this recess forms the auditory (pharyngo-tympanic; Eustachian) tube, and also the tympanic (middle ear) cavity. The pharyngeal arch cartilages are also associated with the development of the ear; it has already been mentioned that their dorsal extremities develop into the middle ear ossicles, the malleus, incus and stapes. A transverse section through the hind-brain during the development of the ear (Fig. 119) shows that the first

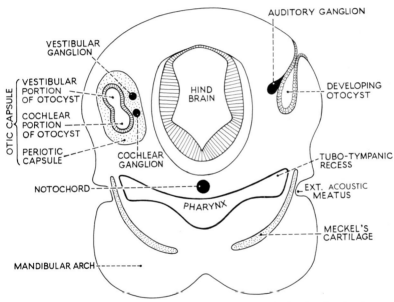

Fig. 119. Diagrammatic transverse section through the hind-brain showing the structures which participate in the development of the vestibulocochlear organ. The dorsal aspect of Meckel's cartilage is seen to be lying in between the endoderm of the tubotympanic recess and the ectoderm of the external acoustic meatus. The developing otocyst is shown on the right of the figure, and the otic capsule on the left, with its constituent parts.

pharyngeal cleft lies immediately lateral to the floor of the outer aspect of the tubo-tympanic recess and develops into the external acoustic meatus. The third and fourth pharyngeal clefts (and usually also the second) become depressed from the surface as the cervical sinus which normally soon becomes obliterated.

The external acoustic meatus is therefore formed from ectoderm and its inner aspect is in contact with the endoderm of the recess; where they are in contact the tympanic membrane is formed but in between the ectoderm and endoderm is the dorsal end of Meckel's cartilage, which develops into the malleus, and a thin layer of mesoderm which produces the fibrous tissue of the membrane. The ectoderm of the membrane forms stratified squamous epithelium on its external aspect and the endoderm of the recess the columnar epithelium on its inner surface. Another structure which is concerned with the development of the vestibulocochlear organ is the *otocyst* (Fig. 120). This is produced as a diverticulum from the ectoderm lateral to

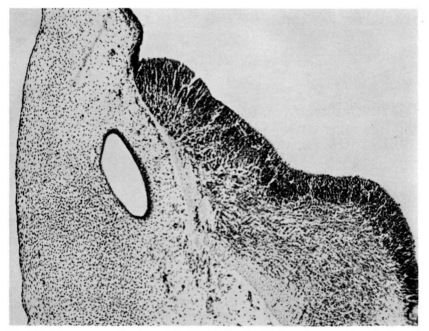

Fig. 120. A transverse section through the hind-brain of an 11·2 mm human embryo to show the otocyst lying immediately lateral to the alar lamina. The dorsal part of the alar lamina is the rhombic lip, and ventral to the alar lamina is the sulcus limitans and basal lamina. ($\times$ 77).

the hind-brain. It grows inwards, becomes cut off from the surface ectoderm and is surrounded by condensed mesoderm, which is called the periotic capsule; this, together with the otocyst, is known as the *otic capsule*.

The internal ear

The otocyst itself develops into the internal ear and becomes divided into a dorsal or vestibular part, and a ventral or cochlear part; from the vestibular part the semicircular canals develop as diverticula. Bast, Anson and Gardner (1947) recognize three main derivatives of the otocyst: (1) the *endolymphatic sac* (a large structure which overlaps the lateral sinus), (2) the utricle with its semicircular canals (the vestibular part), and (3) the saccule with its prolongation, the cochlear duct. The cochlear duct becomes extremely tortuous and forms the cochlea of the adult but only the scala media of the cochlea, the scalae tympani and vestibuli being produced as a result of rarefaction in the periotic capsule (see Streeter, 1917). Coincidentally, there is a proliferation of cells, which differentiate into neuroblasts, from the wall of the otocyst (Politzer, 1956; Batten, 1958) to form a large ganglionic mass, the vestibulocochlear ("auditory" or "acoustic"; Fig. 119) ganglion, closely associated with the otocyst. This ganglion later becomes related to the sensory ganglion of the facial nerve; so close is this relationship that earlier workers considered the two ganglia to develop together from the neural crest as the acoustico-facial ganglion. It is now known, however, that the geniculate ganglion remains independent from the start and comes to lie on the genu of the facial nerve inside the petrous part of the temporal bone, formed by chondrification and eventual endochondral ossification of the periotic capsule. Deol (1967, 1970), has claimed that in mice showing a genetic defect known as "piebald-lethal" and also in white cats and piebald dogs there are defects in the inner ear which suggest that the "acoustic" ganglion in these animals is derived from the neural crest in large part, as well as from the otic placode or otocyst and that these findings are applicable to man and all mammals.

When the otocyst becomes divided into vestibular and cochlear parts, the vestibulocochlear ganglion also divides to form the vestibular and cochlear ganglia, which become associated with the two parts of the otocyst. The internal ear developed from the otocyst (Fig. 121) lies dorsal to the pharynx. The third pharyngeal arch and its contained structures lie immediately behind the tubotympanic recess. The artery of this arch and its continuation, the internal carotid artery (Fig. 121), passes on to the dorsal aspect of the pharynx. In describing the development of the tongue, it was mentioned that the third arch tends to grow forwards; in doing so it constricts the lumen of the tubotympanic recess in its proximal part so that only the outer part of it remains dilated as the tympanic cavity, the proximal constricted part of it forming the auditory tube (Frazer, 1914). The chorda tympani nerve is also found in this situation, since it runs forwards into the first arch over the roof of the first pharyngeal pouch, and therefore comes to be included within the tympanic membrane lying medial to the handle of the malleus.

The internal carotid artery as it is lying dorsal to the pharynx gives off the remains of the second pharyngeal arch artery, which runs laterally and perforates the dorsal end of Reichert's cartilage; the latter forms the stapes which is perforated by the artery. When the artery itself degenerates the place of perforation in Reichert's cartilage remains as a hole in the stapes, which therefore achieves its characteristic adult shape; the artery is therefore called *the stapedial artery*. The malleus and chorda tympani nerve are caught in between the ectoderm of the first pharyngeal cleft and the endoderm of the first pharyngeal pouch and therefore lie in the substance of the tympanic membrane.

In the larval amblystoma (axolotl) normal differentiation of the ears is dependent upon the intactness of the medulla oblongata (Detwiler, 1948, 1951; Detwiler and van Dyke, 1950) and even when the embryonic mid-brain is replaced experimentally by a supernumerary medulla the otic placodes show a remarkable degree of differentiation provided they are grafted along with the medulla, despite their heterotopic position (Detwiler, 1949).

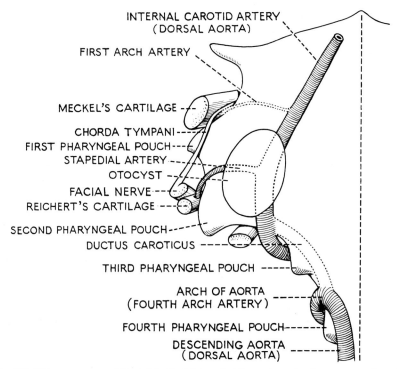

INTERNAL CAROTID ARTERY
(DORSAL AORTA)
FIRST ARCH ARTERY
MECKEL'S CARTILAGE
CHORDA TYMPANI
FIRST PHARYNGEAL POUCH
STAPEDIAL ARTERY
OTOCYST
FACIAL NERVE
REICHERT'S CARTILAGE
SECOND PHARYNGEAL POUCH
DUCTUS CAROTICUS
THIRD PHARYNGEAL POUCH
ARCH OF AORTA
(FOURTH ARCH ARTERY)
FOURTH PHARYNGEAL POUCH
DESCENDING AORTA
(DORSAL AORTA)

Fig. 121. The appearance of the left half of the roof of the embryonic pharynx, seen from the dorsal aspect to show the relations of the otocyst. Modified from Frazer (1910).

The derivatives of pharyngeal pouches

Other structures as well as the auditory tube and the tympanic cavity arise from the pharyngeal pouches. The second pouch is the site of formation of the tonsil; the growth of the third arch mesoderm forwards surrounds the second pouch and forms the tissue of the tonsil, while the second pouch forms the intra-tonsillar cleft. It has been claimed, however (see Hamilton and Hinsch, 1957), that the second pouch leaves no derivatives in the adult. From the third pouch are developed two structures, from the dorsal aspect one of the parathyroids on each side and from the ventral aspect the thymus. The undifferentiated embryonic epithelial thymic cells develop into both the reticular-epithelial cells of the organ parenchyma and lymphoblasts (Ackerman and Knouff, 1964). In this situation, therefore, lymphocytes in the thymus are derived from endoderm rather than mesoderm. In the adult, thymus derived lymphocytes (T cells) have quite different immunological functions to those derived from lymph nodes (B lymphocytes).

A parathyroid also develops from each fourth pouch. The parathyroids which develop from the third pouches form the inferior pair of parathyroids. This is due to the fact that the thymus which also develops from the third pouch becomes attached on to the arch of the aorta during development and as the heart "descends" it takes with it the arch of the aorta, and therefore the thymus, which in turn pulls down the third pouch parathyroids to a lower level than those developed from the fourth pouch.

The *ultimobranchial body* is a structure which develops from the fifth pouch; this together with the fourth pouch is termed the *fourth pouch complex*. It was thought at one time to form the lateral lobes of the thyroid gland but this is now known to be untrue, since all of the follicles of the thyroid develop in man from the diverticulum from the floor of the pharynx (p. 224). Although the ultimobranchial body does become applied to the inferior pole of the lateral lobe of the thyroid gland during development, it develops into cells within the thyroid gland which differ from thyroid follicular cells (see Boyd, 1950; Bejdl and Politzer, 1953). It is now known that the cells within the thyroid gland which develop from the ultimobranchial body are the parafollicular "light" or C cells, which are concerned with the secretion of *calcitonin,* a hypocalcaemic hormone (see Hirsch and Manson, 1969). The likelihood of adenomata and carcinomata arising from such remains of ultimobranchial tissue must not be overlooked (van Dyke, 1945). Thymic tissue may develop from the fourth pouch and the pharyngeal region as a whole has the potentiality for developing thymus and parathyroid tissue, so that parathyroids may develop from thymus and thymus from parathyroid or thyroid tissue. There is therefore a slight possibility of thyroid tissue developing from the fourth pharyngeal pouch or the ultimobranchial body (Kingsbury, 1939). The ultimobranchial body remains as a separate gland in fish, amphibia and birds and only fuses with the thyroid gland in mammals. Extracts of the body from these lower vertebrates have a hypocalcaemic activity in rats. Most incongruous, however, is the fact that this activity also resides in the ultimobranchial tissue of sharks, which are non-bony fish.

CLINICAL RELATIONSHIPS

Abnormalities of the visual apparatus

If the distal part of the hyaloid artery persists, it may interfere with vision, just like a persistent pupillary membrane. Opacities of the lens (congenital cataract) are common in children whose mothers had Rubella during the second month of pregnancy. There is a high incidence in Down's Syndrome. If the hyaloid fissure fails to close, there is an absence of a sector of the iris, which may include the ciliary body, retina or choroid; this is a defect known as typical coloboma, the absent sector being directed downwards.

An eye may be absent (anophthalmia) or small (microphthalmia), or the lens alone may fail to develop (aphakia). At an earlier stage of development, if the optic centres fail to undergo paired organization, a single, median eye results (cyclopia) and, of course, there are all grades of degrees of approximation of the two eyes.

The eyelids may fail to separate before birth (ankyloblepharon). In severe cases, the skin passes continuously from the brow over the eye to the cheek (cryptophthalmia). Coloboma may also occur in the eyelids, usually in the upper eyelid and is generally manifest as a notch in the edge of the lid to the inner side of the midline. Distichiasis is a rare disorder in which there are two rows of cilia, often in all four lids.

In an *arrest* of development (Mann, 1957), such as failure of formation of the optic vesicle, a condition of anophthalmia will be produced in which the retina, ciliary and iris epithelium and optic nerve are absent. Lack of organizer activity from the optic vesicle means that the lens also fails to develop. The mesodermal elements of the eye (choroid, sclera, extrinsic muscles, conjunctiva, lids and orbit) will, however, develop, although smaller than normal, since they are self-determining. Complete absence of the iris (aniridia) is similarly an arrest of development. In anomalies arising as a result of *aberration* of development, the abnormal growth may be an overgrowth (e.g. spreading of myelin sheaths of optic nerve fibres on to the retina, when they should stop at the lamina cribrosa), or an abnormal development that resembles no stage normal in man or other animals (e.g. atypical coloboma of the iris, in which the absent sector of the iris occurs anywhere in its circumference and does not involve the ciliary body). The greater proportion of all gross abnormalities of the eye are, however, produced by arrest followed by aberration of development. An example is microphthalmia with cyst formation, in which the eye resembles that at an earlier age, but with an added cystic structure attached. A congenital cystic eye is produced by arrest of development before complete invagination of the optic vesicle. If oxygen is administered to babies with apnoea or hypoxia, there is a danger of producing retrolental fibroplasia.

Maternal rubella occurring between the second and third months of pregnancy, is often followed by defective development of the eyes, ears and heart. If the mother is infected at about the 6th week of pregnancy, the growth of primary lens fibres in the lens vesicle is affected and a *nuclear cataract* of the lens occurs. If the infection occurs at eight or nine weeks, the lens escapes but the child may be born deaf as a result of imperfect differentiation of the organ of Corti in the cochlea.

Ear anomalies

Congenital deafness may also result from abnormal development of the tympanic membrane or the middle ear ossicles; the VIIIth nerve may also fail to develop normally. Atresia of the external acoustic meatus or of the auditory tube and tympanic cavity may result from defective development of the first pharyngeal cleft or the first pouch respectively. Since the auricle develops as six hillocks of tissue around the first cleft, retarded development may result in a persistence of the embryonic or fetal condition, when there are resultant clefts or pits between the tragus and antitragus, or in the helix.

Thyroid anomalies

Abnormality in descent of the thyroid gland during development may result in the presence of thyroid tissue in the tongue—a lingual thyroid—or at the other extreme, a retrosternal thyroid. Indeed, thyroid tissue may form anywhere along the course of the thyroglossal duct. More common, however, is a thyroglossal cyst. Since, when the cyst is removed surgically, as much as possible of the duct is also extirpated, the relationship of the duct to the hyoid bone is important; because the body of the hyoid develops from second and third arches, the duct must clearly lie anterior to the hyoid. Occasionally the two lateral lobes of the thyroid are unequal in size and one lobe may rarely be absent. The isthmus may be absent or fused with one or other lobe. In about 40% cases there is a pyramidal lobe, a process of the isthmus upwards towards the hyoid, usually to one side of the midline. Occasionally the myoblasts of the part of the rectus column in the neck which forms the thyrohyoid muscle extend downwards during development to become attached to the pyramidal lobe as the levator glandulae thyroidae.

The pyramidal lobe probably represents aberrant thyroid tissue development from the lower end of the thyroglossal duct. Complete absence (agenesia) of the thyroid leads to congenital cretinism, a condition characterized by stunted mental and physical development and a typical bloated facial appearance.

References

Ackerman, G. A. and Knouff, R. A. (1964). Lymphocyte formation in the thymus of the embryonic chick. *Anat. Rec.* **149**, 191-216.

Amprino, R. (1951). Developmental correlations between the eye and associated structures. *J. exp. Zool.* **118**, 71-100.

Bast, T. H., Anson, B. J. and Gardner, W. D. (1947). Developmental course of the human auditory vesicle. *Anat. Rec.* **99**, 55-74.

Batten, E. H. (1958). The origin of the acoustic ganglion in the sheep. *J. Embryol. exp. Morph.* **6**, 597-615.

Bejdl, W. and Politzer, G. (1953). Über die Frühentwicklung des telobranchialen Körpers beim Menschen. *Z. Anat. EntwGesch.* **117**, 136-152.

Boyd, J. D. (1950). Development of the thyroid and parathyroid glands and the thymus. *Ann. R. C. Surg. Eng.* **7**, 455-471.

Deol, M. S. (1967). The neural crest and the acoustic ganglion. *J. Embryol. exp. Morph.* **17,** 533-541.

Deol, M. S. (1970). The origin of the acoustic ganglion and effects of the gene dominant spotting (Wv) in the mouse. *J. Embryol. exp. Morph.* **23,** 773-784.

Detwiler, S. R. (1948). Further quantitative studies on locomotor capacity of larval ambystoma following surgical procedures on the adult brain. *J. exp. Zool.* **108,** 45-74.

Detwiler, S. R. (1949). The responses of ambystoma larvae with the midbrain replaced by a supernumerary medulla. *J. exp. Zool.* **110,** 321-335.

Detwiler, S. R. (1951). Further experimental observations on the differentation of the otic vesicle in ambystoma. *J. exp. Zool.* **116,** 415-430.

Detwiler, S. R. and Van Dyke, R. H. (1950). The role of the medulla in the differentiation of the otic vesicle. *J. exp. Zool.* **113,** 179-200.

Dyke, J. H. van (1945). Behaviour of ultimobranchial tissue in the postnatal thyroid gland: epithelial cysts, their relation to thyroid parenchyma and to "new growths" in the thyroid gland of young sheep. *Amer. J. Anat.* **76,** 201-252.

Frazer, J. E. (1910). The early development of the eustachian tube and pharynx. *Br. med. J.* **ii,** 1148-1151.

Frazer, J. E. (1914). The second visceral arch and groove in the tubo-tympanic region. *J. Anat.* **48,** 391-408.

Hamilton, H. L. and Hinsch, G. W. (1957). The fate of the second visceral pouch in the chick. *Anat. Rec.* **129,** 357-370.

Hirsch, P. F. and Manson, P. L. (1969). Thyrocalcitonin. *Physiol. Rev.* **49,** 548-622.

Kingsbury, B. F. (1939). The question of a lateral thyroid in mammals with special reference to man. *Am. J. Anat.* **65,** 333-360.

Mann, I. (1949). "The Development of the Human Eye" British Medical Association, London.

Mann, I. (1957). "Developmental Abnormalities of the Eye" British Medical Association, London.

Planel, H. (1951). "Etudes Anatomiques et Physiologiques sur les Fosses nasales des Rongeurs" R. Lion et Fils, Toulouse.

Politzer, G. (1956). Die entstehung des ganglion acusticum beim menschen. *Acta Anat.* **26,** 1-13.

Sheppard, T. H., Andersen, H. J. and Andersen, H. (1964a). The human fetal thyroid. I. Its weight in relation to body weight, crown-rump length, foot length and estimated gestation age. *Anat. Rec.* **148,** 123.

Sheppard, T. H., Andersen, H. and Andersen, H. J. (1964b). Histochemical studies of the human fetal thyroid during the first half of fetal life. *Anat. Rec.* **149,** 363-380.

Streeter, G. L. (1917). The factors involved in the excavation of the cavities in the cartilaginous capsule of the ear in the human embryo. *Am. J. Anat.* **22,** 1-25.

22

The Development of the Suprarenal Gland

Development of cortex and medulla

The cortex of the suprarenal gland develops as a proliferation of cells first from the coelomic epithelium (splanchnopleuric intraembryonic mesoderm) in the medial coelomic bay and later from the glomerular capsules of the mesonephros (Crowder, 1957). This forms a swelling (Fig. 122) lying medial to the mesonephros, and also therefore in close relationship to the gonadal ridge. The swelling becomes invaded on its dorsomedial border by cells which have migrated from the neural crest; these cells differentiate into the medulla of the gland.

The cortex developing in early fetal life (the *fetal cortex*) is later covered on its external aspect by another mass of cells which proliferate from the splanchnopleuric intraembryonic mesoderm and this forms the true adult suprarenal cortex. The fetal cortex degenerates after birth but until this time it remains as a zone of cells lying between the adult suprarenal cortex and the medulla. This is probably not identical with the "X-zone" which is in a similar position in mice and was once termed the "androgenic zone" since it was believed to secrete androgenic hormones (Grollman, 1933) although there is no sound evidence for such a belief. Broster and Vines (1933) found a fuchsinophil substance in suprarenal cortical cells of the male fetus between the tenth and seventeenth weeks of gestation and in the female fetus only between the eleventh and fifteenth weeks and claim that virilism (masculinization) of suprarenal origin is related to this "male phase" of suprarenal cortical development. Although fuchsinophilia may demonstrate the number and distribution of mitochondria in suprarenal cortical cells (see Cain and Harrison, 1950), it does not specifically detect the presence of androgens.

At birth, the suprarenal gland is relatively undifferentiated but, nevertheless, larger in relation to the size of the kidney than in postnatal life. The gland only reaches its complete development at puberty (Frazao, 1954), the time when the zona reticularis is formed. The medulla is rudimentary at birth and only achieves full development at age 22 months postnatally. Production of cortical cells continues into postnatal life (see Cain and Harrison, 1950) and in this respect, as also in relation to the histochemistry of the suprarenal cortex, the zona glomerulosa appears to be functionally separate from the other two zones.

Since the cells of the suprarenal medulla develop from neural crest tissue, they are themselves post-ganglionic sympathetic neurons and therefore the sympathetic nerves innervating the medulla are pre-ganglionic. Because of the different origin of the medulla, it has its own blood supply (the arteriae medullae); the close association of the cortex and medulla, however, ensures that the three hormones secreted by the medulla can alter the distribution of blood flowing through the gland (Harrison and Hoey, 1960; Harrison and Brown, 1964). In similar fashion, stimulation of sympathetic nerves to the gland can affect the vascularization of the cortex (Brown and Harrison, 1964).

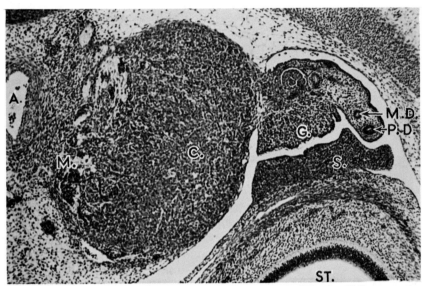

Fig. 122. Photomicrograph of the developing suprarenal cortex (C.) of a 17·5 mm human embryo. Neural crest cells are infiltrating the dorsomedial border of the cortex to produce suprarenal medullary tissue (M.). Lying lateral to the suprarenal may be seen the developing gonad (G.) and the mesonephric (M.D.) and paramesonephric (P.D.) ducts. The aorta (A.), spleen (S.) and stomach (ST.) are also visible. (× 77).

CLINICAL RELATIONSHIPS

Suprarenal cortical hyperplasia, with its consequent augmentation of hormonal secretion, can produce virilism—a phenomenon of masculinization, including enlargement of the clitoris and growth of hair on the face—in adult women, or feminization in adult men. In fetal life or, to a lesser extent in prepubertal life, this disorder can have far more profound consequences, by the production of *pseudohermaphroditism,* an abnormality in which the person has the gonads of one sex but a varying degree of tendency towards the development of external genitalia of the opposite sex (see p. 176). The male pseudohermaphrodite has a normal XY chromosomal constitution and may have external genitalia which are entirely female in appearance, is reared as a female and at puberty feminises well with good breast development and female secondary sexual characteristics;

he may marry and have normal sexual relationships but cannot bear children because he does not possess a uterus. The testes are usually present but undescended in the inguinal region. The other type of male pseudohermaphrodite has male or partly masculinized (ambiguous) genitalia and the testes may have descended into the inguinal region or even a cleft scrotum. Hypospadias and a vagina or even a uterus may be present. He may either masculinize or feminize at puberty. Female pseudohermaphrodites have an XX chromosome constitution and normal ovaries. There are varying degrees of masculinization of the external genitalia, but a uterus and uterine tubes are always present. A scrotum may be present and the urogenital sinus may persist with a single external orifice. The clitoris is enlarged to the extent that occasionally a well-developed penis may be present. Other defects such as imperforate anus and anomalies of the urinary tract may accompany this disorder.

Some individuals with the clinical characteristics of male pseudo-hermaphroditism are, in fact, mosaics such as XO/XY, XO/XXY and show abnormal development of the gonads; they should therefore properly be considered as cases of gonadal dysgenesis.

In some cases of anencephaly, there is an associated defect in the development of the pituitary gland. This is accompanied by a defective development of the cortex of the suprarenal. Nodules of accessory supra-renal cortical tissue are frequently found normally in the tissue surrounding the suprarenals or in the perinephric fat. Occasionally, nodules of accessory cortical tissue are found within the spermatic cord or even in the testis itself. These nodules enlarge considerably following suprarenalectomy. The collection of suprarenal cortex together with accessory cortical tissue warrants the concept of a "cortical system" which reacts as a whole in response to stress. The chromaffin system is similarly to be considered as the collection of separate masses of chromaffin tissue in the body including both the suprarenal medulla and the widely distributed extra-suprarenal chromaffin bodies, particularly the para-aortic bodies and the entero-chromaffin cells in the wall of the intestine. The para-aortic bodies become dispersed soon after birth; by puberty they are hardly visible to the naked eye. Their regression is roughly paralleled by the maturation of the suprarenal medulla.

Since the suprarenal glands develop in close relation to the mesonephroi, the left gland utilizes the inter-subcardinal anastomosis for its venous drainage, whilst the right drains into the inferior vena cava. The right suprarenal vein is consequently very much shorter than the left, little more than a diverticulum of the I.V.C. For this and other reasons, surgical removal of the right gland is much more difficult. Since the suprarenals are much larger in fetal life, they become extensively vascularized by lateral branches of the aorta; in the adult, although the gland is vascularized from three main sources, the inferior phrenic artery, the renal artery and a branch direct from the aorta, there may be a total of as many as 50 separate arteries supplying each suprarenal. Each artery is an end-artery to the zona fasciculata of the cortex.

References

Broster, L. R. and Vines, H. W. C. (1933). "The Adrenal Cortex" H. K. Lewis, London.

Brown, K. N. and Harrison, R. G. (1964). The effect of sympathetic nerve stimulation on suprarenal cortical vascularization in the rat. *J. Anat.* **98**, 11-16.

Cain, A. J. and Harrison, R. G. (1950). Cytological and histochemical variations in the adrenal cortex of the albino rat. *J. Anat.* **84**, 196-226.

Crowder, R. E. (1957). The development of the adrenal gland in man, with special reference to origin and ultimate location of cell types and evidence in favour of cell "migration" theory. *Contr. Embryol.* **36**, 193-210.

Frazao, J. Vasconcelos (1954). "A Glândula Córtico-suprarrenal" Livraria Portugalia, Lisbon.

Grollman, A. (1936). "The Adrenals" Balliere, Tindall & Cox, London.

Harrison, R. G. and Brown, K. N. (1964). Suprarenal cortical degeneration following isoproterenol administration in the rat. *Endocrinology* **75**, 173-178.

Harrison, R. G. and Hoey, M. J. (1960). "The Adrenal Circulation" Blackwell Scientific Publications, Oxford.

23

Regeneration

It was stressed in the Introduction to this book that development is not the prerogative of the prenatal period of life, since it continues in the postnatal phase. It has already been noted that some organs are not even fully developed at birth; the reproductive system, because it is normally inactive until "puberty", is typically late in developing and, indeed, the mammary gland (p. 71) and prostate (p. 169) are very immature at birth. In adult life, in addition, tissues have considerable powers of regeneration.

Regeneration is the repair by growth and differentiation of damage suffered by an organism past the phase of primordial development (Weiss, 1939). Regenerative processes are fundamentally of the same nature and follow the same principles as the ontogenetic processes. The capacity for regeneration is not a secondarily acquired adeptness at meeting later damage by adequate repair but is a residue of the original capacity for growth, organization and differentiation. The extent of regenerative capacity is therefore dependent upon the extent of survival of developmental capacity during ontogenesis.

There is a general impression that the capacity for regeneration is less the greater the degree of organization. This is mostly true; but, in specific instances, it is often extremely difficult to predict an animal's capacity for regeneration from its position phylogenetically. Within a given species, also, the cells of some tissues have more regenerative capacity than others and it is in such tissues as skin, connective tissue, bone, skeletal muscle and blood, in which proliferation of new cells continues markedly into postnatal life to repair loss of tissue through wear and tear, that regenerative capacity is clearly observable. Yet some tissues which are often considered to be highly organized, such as liver and the axons of peripheral nerves, have immense powers of regeneration.

There are similar variations in the response of tissues to damaging influences, such as ischaemia. In general, organs of endodermal origin, such as the stomach, intestine, thyroid, urinary bladder and pancreas appear to withstand ischaemia fairly well, probably because their arterial supply is provided with particularly rich arterial anastomoses; but organs and tissues developed from mesoderm and ectoderm vary considerably in their reaction to ischaemia produced by the interruption of individual arteries of supply.

Powers of regeneration also depend on the extent of damage. Replacement of a complete organ in mammals, for example the adult human liver, is impossible and death rapidly ensues after complete hepatectomy but after partial hepatectomy of even threequarters of the liver substance, complete regeneration of the whole organ can occur. Certain cells in a tissue may also show different regenerative powers when compared with others. Thus connective tissue has excellent powers of regeneration, for example in repairing a skin wound, but the fat cells in it do not appear to have a good regenerative capacity in the adult, since if a localized pad of fat is partially removed there is no compensatory hypertrophy of the remainder, although fat cells are derived from connective tissue cells indistinguishable mor- phologically from fibroblasts (see Clark, 1971). The fat cell presumably possesses a higher degree of cellular organization than the fibroblast and is less plastic in its functions in addition. In this respect cellular differentiation has progressed to a degree completely incompatible with mitosis, since the multifarious functions and potentialities of a fibroblast have become suppressed and subservient to the sole function of fat storage important to a fat cell.

Regeneration of whole organs can, however, take place in lower vertebrates (see Chalkley, 1959). Regenerative capacity is great in amphibian larvae, which can regenerate whole eyes, limbs or a tail for example. Even the adult newt, *Triturus v. viridescens,* is able to regenerate its iris and lens (see Stone and Griffith, 1954; Stone, 1955, 1957), a process impossible in mammals, since the iris is produced developmentally from the optic cup, an outgrowth from the brain and the mammalian central nervous system which have very poor powers of regeneration.

During the repair of a defect in certain organs or tissues, the cells involved are often not the organ-specific cells but less organized cells such as fibroblasts. In the repair process, cell dedifferentiation has occurred and the existence of this phenomenon depends on various factors such as the degree of differentiation achieved in the organ concerned and the extent of damage. Thus, cardiac muscle is incapable of regeneration (Harrison, 1947) in mammals, but regeneration can occur to the extent of repairing a very limited destruction of rabbit skeletal muscle (Clark, 1946). In human skeletal muscles, however, fibrosis in areas of local destruction proceeds so rapidly as to prevent significant regeneration of muscle fibres and such rapid fibrosis may also be one of the factors responsible for the lack of regeneration of cardiac muscle. This phenomenon can be seen in many tissues, such as an area of focal necrosis in the zona fasciculata of the suprarenal cortex caused by ischaemia (Harrison, 1951). It may also be responsible, in a modified form resulting from overproduction of neuroglial tissue (see Windle, 1956), for the poor regenerative capacity of central nervous system axons. Indeed, ischaemic tissue generally, because of lack of oxygen and nutrition, commonly shows dedifferentiation and only in the presence of adequate collateral circulation can regeneration occur.

In certain tissues such as cartilage, specific cells are responsible for postnatal growth. In the regeneration of cartilage perichondrial cells are responsible, though these cells are at first indistinguishable from fibroblasts. Localized pressure and friction may also lead to the production of cartilage by metaplasia of ordinary connective tissue elements and this is strong evidence that cartilage formation is not necessarily dependent on specific chondroblasts (Clark, 1971).

Apart from an adequate blood supply and nutrition, nervous impulses are essential for the regeneration of many tissues. Mechanical forces are also necessary for the orientation of some tissues (e.g. tendon) during regeneration; this is only one of many factors which may influence the organization of regenerating tissue and the resumption of its functional activity. Some of these factors (e.g. age, temperature) may, in addition, affect tissue survival before regeneration commences.

Direct redevelopment *in situ* of a portion lost, as in the limbs of crustacea and amphibia, has been termed "epimorphosis" in contrast to "morphallaxis" in which the remaining portion of the body is remodelled to restore the whole form (see Needham, 1952). Related to morphallaxis, in the sense that the initial form is not restored precisely, is "compensatory hypertrophy", as in the regeneration of the liver and other internal organs; it is probably a response to functional demands. This, and other aspects of regeneration, are discussed by Goss (1964). Wound healing is an epimorphic process on a small scale and involves regressive and progressive phases. In the regressive phase damaged cells are removed and there is tissue reaction to the damaging influence; dedifferentiation, if it occurs, should probably be included in this phase. In the progressive phase, growth and differentiation of the regenerating tissues takes place. This phase may be more complicated in some tissues, for example regenerating liver, in which a period of rapid regeneration is followed by a period of alternating focal necrosis (localized cell death) and regeneration (Wilson *et al.,* 1953). As in ontogeny, regenerated structures function before reaching their definitive size and function probably promotes hypertrophy and hyperplasia of the regenerating tissues.

Dempster (1957) discusses wound healing and the stimulus which evokes repair of a wound. He shows that there are many factors involved in this process and demonstrates that no one trophic stimulus or hormone can be considered responsible. Nevertheless, in certain instances, such as the regeneration of a peripheral nerve fibre or skeletal muscle fibre, the organization of specific cells (neurilemmal cells + endoneurium or sarcolemmal cells + endomysium respectively around the regenerating axon or sarcoplasm) appears to be essential.

In general, exposed parts of animals regenerate best (Lessona's rule). Skin regeneration in man is most effective but, as already noted, some mammalian internal organs such as the liver are able to regenerate efficiently, and this may be an enhanced response to wear and tear, an exaggeration of the mechanism of compensatory hypertrophy.

The nucleic acids of ribonucleoprotein (R.N.A.) and deoxyribonucleoprotein (D.N.A.) are intimately concerned in the regenerative powers of cells (see Needham, 1952). D.N.A. is localized primarily in the chromosomes, although it is also found in mitochondria and other self-reproducing organelles. Its polynucleotide molecule is arranged as a double helix. D.N.A. is the hereditary material, being capable of replication (self-duplication) under the influence of the enzyme D.N.A. polymerase. The bulk of the R.N.A. of a cell is found in the cytoplasm, although some is found in the nucleus (about 10% in mammals), primarily in the nucleolus, with smaller amounts on the chromosomes and in the nuclear sap. It seems that the sole role of the single stranded R.N.A. molecules in the cell is with protein synthesis and most of this synthesis takes place in the cytoplasm. Further, it appears that D.N.A. is involved in the synthesis of R.N.A. Under the influence of the enzyme R.N.A. polymerase working off one of the strands of the D.N.A. double helix, "messenger" R.N.A. is synthesized in the nucleus and then passes into the cytoplasm to become attached to ribosomes. In like manner another type of R.N.A., "transfer" R.N.A., is also synthesized in the nucleus from D.N.A.; this acts as an "adaptor" (or connector) between cytoplasmic amino acids and the messenger R.N.A., so constituting the first steps in protein synthesis. Since each molecule of transfer R.N.A. is specific for a given amino acid, specific proteins can be built up in the cell. Some of the R.N.A. synthesized in the nucleus stays there and is concerned with nucleoprotein synthesis.

In this way it can be seen that larger molecules of the cell are built up from smaller molecules. The larger molecules, be they proteins, nucleic acids or lipids, in turn come together with each other or with other similar molecules to form a complex protein system acting as an enzyme, a multienzyme complex, or a D.N.A. complex, and so on. In turn, these larger aggregates interact with one another to form structures such as membranes (mostly lipid and protein), ribosomes (mostly R.N.A. and protein) or chromosomes (mostly D.N.A. and protein). In this way, cellular structure is built up and regulated and it is clear that such processes as those described above are involved in both the regeneration of cells and the growth of daughter cells during mitosis, as well as in spermatogenesis, oogenesis and the cleavage of the fertilized ovum. The description of cellular dynamics outlined above is only a brief and very inadequate summary of the complex processes which have been observed to occur in recent years; Loewy and Siekevitz (1969) should be consulted for a more authoritative description of cellular biology at the molecular level.

Cells from most individuals are proficient in the repair of D.N.A. damage. Retrospective studies have shown that individuals defective in repair are cancer prone and our knowledge of the molecular nature of the defects leads to the strong prediction that unrepaired damage to D.N.A. has a high carcinogenic potential (Setlow, 1978). The complexity of carcinogenesis, on the other hand, also indicates that not all cancers arise from defects in repair. Nevertheless, even in normal individuals the rate of D.N.A. repair compared with other cellular processes should be an important parameter in the initial steps in carcinogenesis. Hence, an understanding of the control and kinetics of repair processes is as important as a knowledge of the activation and inactivation pathways for chemical carcinogens in extrapolations of carcinogenic hazards to humans.

These cellular features demonstrate that the metabolic processes involved in regeneration have many similarities with those occurring during human ontogenesis, further evidence that development continues from prenatal into postnatal periods, and that man should be studied in his entirety rather than in isolated compartments of embryology and anatomy.

References

Chalkley, D. T. (1959). *In* "Regeneration in Vertebrates" Ed. C. S. Thornton. Chap. III, p. 34. Univ. of Chicago Press.

Clark, W. E. Le Gros (1946). The regeneration of mammalian striped muscle. *J. Anat.* **80**, 24-36.

Clark, W. E. Le Gros (1971). "The Tissues of the Body" 6th. Edn. Clarendon Press, Oxford.

Dempster, W. J. (1957). "An Introduction to Experimental Surgical Studies" Blackwell Scientific Publications, Oxford.

Goss, R. J. (1964). "Adaptive Growth" Logos Press, London.

Harrison, R. G. (1947). The regenerative capacity of cardiac muscle. *J. Anat.* **81**, 365-366.

Harrison, R. G. (1951). A comparative study of the vascularization of the adrenal gland in the rabbit, rat and cat. *J. Anat.* **85**, 12-23.

Loewy, A. G. and Siekevitz, P. (1969). "Cell Structure and Function" Holt, Rinehart and Winston, London.

Needham, A. E. (1952). "Regeneration and Wound-Healing" Methuen, London.

Setlow, R. B. (1978). Repair deficient human disorders and cancer. *Nature* **271**, 713-717.

Stone, L. S. (1955). Regeneration of the iris and lens from retina pigment cells in adult newt eyes. *J. exp. Zool.* **129**, 505-534.

Stone, L. S. (1957). Regeneration of iris and lens in hypophysectomised adult newts. *J. exp. Zool.* **136**, 17-34.

Stone, L. S. and Griffith, B. H. (1954). Regeneration of the iris and lens in eyes of adult *Triturus v. viridescens. J. exp. Zool.* **127**, 153-180.

Weiss, P. (1939). "Principles of Development" Henry Holt, New York.

Wilson, M. E., Stowell, R. D., Yakoyama, H. O. and Tsuboi, K. K. (1953). Cytological changes in regenerating mouse liver. *Cancer Res.* **13**, 86-92.

Windle, W. F. (1956). Regeneration of axons in the vertebrate central nervous system. *Physiol. Rev.* **36**, 427-440.

INDEX